MW01093973

A Physical Education

A Physical Education

How I Escaped Diet Culture and Gained the Power of Lifting

Casey Johnston

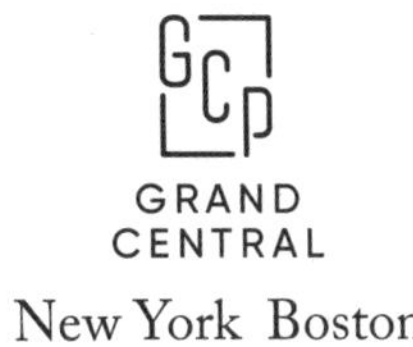

New York Boston

This memoir reflects the author's life faithfully rendered to the best of her ability. Some names and identifying details have been changed to protect the privacy of others. In addition, the diet and exercise information included is not intended to replace the services of trained health professionals, or be a substitute for medical advice. You are advised to consult with your health care professional with regard to matters relating to your health, diet, and exercise.

Cover design by Claire Sullivan

Grand Central Publishing
Hachette Book Group
1290 Avenue of the Americas, New York, NY 10104
grandcentralpublishing.com
@grandcentralpub

First Edition: May 2025

Grand Central Publishing is a division of Hachette Book Group, Inc. The Grand Central Publishing name and logo is a registered trademark of Hachette Book Group, Inc.

Print book interior design by Marie Mundaca

Library of Congress Cataloging-in-Publication Data has been applied for.

ISBNs: 978-1-5387-7325-3 (hardcover); 978-1-5387-7327-7 (ebook)

Printed in the United States of America.

LSC-C

Printing 1, 2025

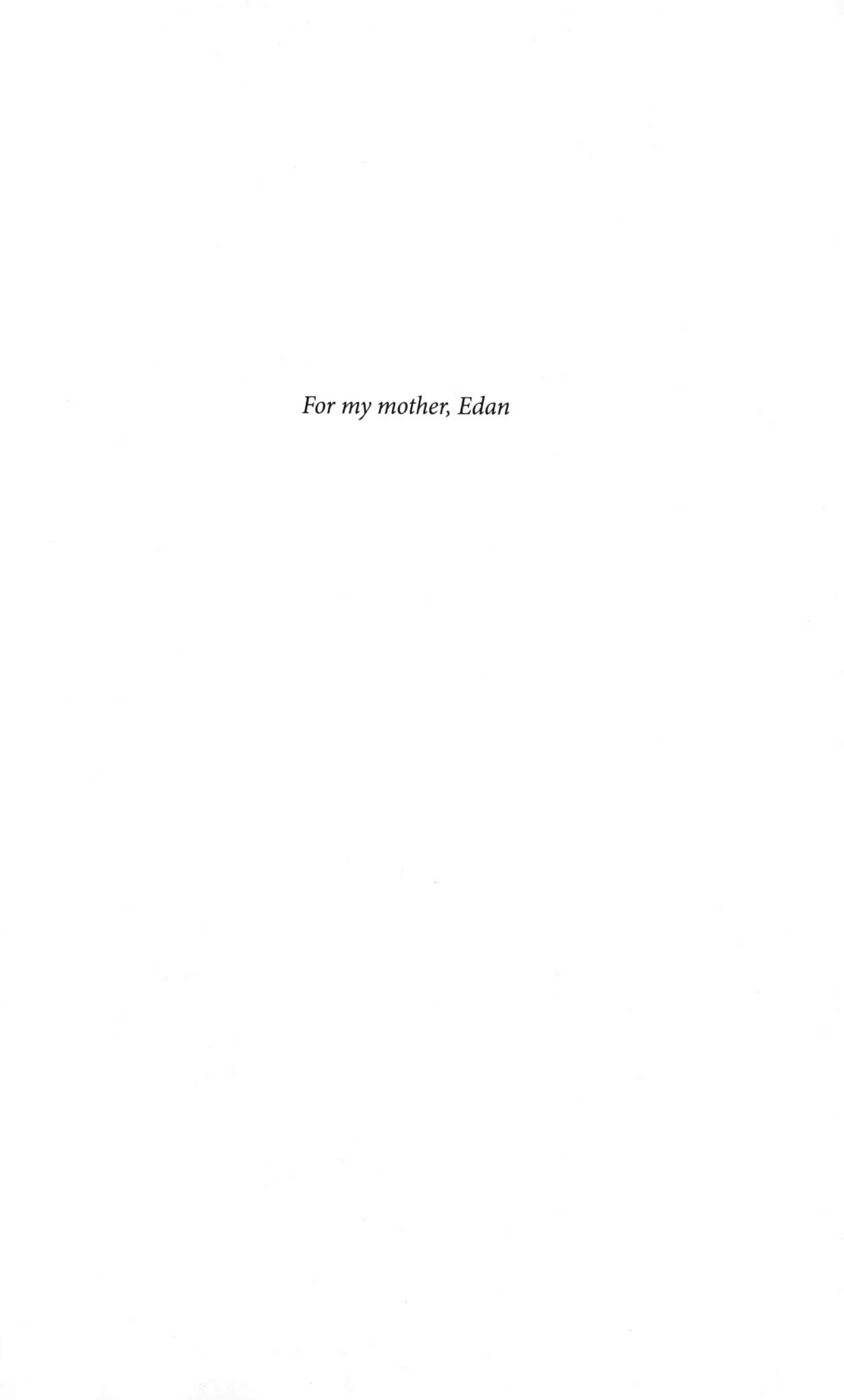

For my mother, Edan

Contents

Contents

Preface

IN 2016, I STARTED writing a science-based, tongue-in-cheek column about lifting weights. To my surprise, a lot of people read it, and before long I was being asked for interviews and invited on podcasts. Inevitably, one question would always come up: What was it about lifting that I loved so much? I would say something along the lines of "It completely changed how I think and feel about the world and myself and everything." I knew that was true, but I didn't know exactly what I meant, and I didn't have the words to put it in more specific terms. This book became about finding those words.

For most of my adult life, I had felt barraged with mandates that I was responsible for following to a T: to lose weight, to burn more calories, to "beat cravings." In more recent years, I understood that lifting weights could change my body functionally, and of course, I'd heard over and over about people who began exercising and benefitted from it. It made them happier, or helped them feel more capable, or gave them a greater sense of control. And sure, lifting weights did make me stronger and I did feel more capable.

But there were other gains I hadn't anticipated. From the first, strength training was emotionally revelatory. I did not expect to discover, over time, that strength could rehabilitate how I shrank from confrontation. Before long, I also had to face my fear of failure. I couldn't help but dive into exploring these effects with my science-reporting chops, and astoundingly came across what research showed: training could change my brain.

It also fascinated me that, instead of pushing answers on me, lifting weights invited me to ask more questions about myself. It began with asking "How did that movement feel, and why?"— two concepts I'd never been prompted to care about before when it came to my body or exercise. Yet this was immediately an instrumental part of customizing lifting workouts to my skill level. Unexpectedly, this basic, atomic practice radiated outward into growing assessments of how I felt in general, which led me to questioning quite a lot. Where did my urgent need to comply with the mandate to lose weight come from? Why did I so often feel avoidant: of confrontation, of family, of risk? Why was I so scared of gyms, afraid of doing unfamiliar activities in front of strangers? Why did I believe it was weird to be strong, that it was reserved for jocks and bros?

In looking for answers, I stumbled upon wide-ranging connecting threads that turned out to inform my many untested opinions about strength, culture, and behavior: from the history of religious culture in America to contemporary media messaging, to the implications of mind-body duality. Closer to home, I even began to reinterpret my role in my family.

All this may be surprising to encounter in a book about lifting weights, a topic that we normally consider surface level—many of us associate it with weight loss, or becoming more beautiful in the conventional sense. For a long time, "weight loss" formed my entire conception of my body. Either I was small enough (and always getting smaller), or I was a disappointment. I'd accepted, as a fact of life, cravings and obsession over my weight and constant stress over how my clothes fit. Wasn't it all pretty simple, even if it was also a continuous, unending drag? There seemed to be no quicker way to undermine everything I cared about or worked at than not delivering on the effort toward appearance that everyone else expected.

But it's hard to recognize how narrow your worldview is until you become receptive to having it challenged. I was no exception.

I felt the differences that came from investing in strength training before I really understood them. The effects took hold quickly, and it felt markedly different, and powerful, to move around in my body. I hadn't realized how much I had been struggling every day, but more importantly, I hadn't realized that the path of *not* struggling had always hovered so close by. I was so used to distrusting myself, and that distrust included my body. Where did that come from? Why had I accepted it for so long, just as a condition of my existence? This question was the foundation from which all of the other changes unfolded.

My personal story forms the scaffolding of this book, and it acts as a springboard from which to build a fresh exposé of diet culture. Diet culture is not just a set of well-intentioned, if sometimes misguided, lifestyle suggestions. Many of its patterns are directly, insidiously harmful, not just psychologically but biologically, in ways that engrave themselves again and again upon our brains and bodies. It's a vicious cycle: the more we participate, the more we become dependent on it, and the more we believe that suffering is a requisite part of our existence (a belief that is itself deeply culturally entrenched). The more I learned about strength, the clearer it became that diet culture is a toxic and dysfunctional wheel that needs to be broken.

But I also use my story to build a scientific and cultural case for building (or rebuilding) strength. Creating strength is actually a process of rupture, rest, and repair: within our cells, as well as metaphorically, within our psyche. It involves becoming attuned inward, getting to know and being generous to ourselves, learning where we are and what we need. I'd always been taught that progress was a matter of raw bravery and grit and willingness to suffer, when, in fact, it requires understanding, self-regard, and patience. It requires respect for our bodies' elegant, interconnected, inextricable systems of muscle, bone, blood, reflex, and memory.

Attributes of my body I'd been taught were distasteful—fat, injury, aches and pains, slowness to respond—only seemed so because I lacked knowledge and understanding. Properly understood and respected as part of a complex system, nothing in a human body is useless or a waste. Not the fat, which protects our organs and our muscles while they recover from illness or exercise; not the body hair, there to protect our skin and block bacteria from our nether regions; not even the trauma, those intrusive thoughts and instinctive reactions that constitute the body's ham-handed attempt to spare us from reruns of past calamity.

And yes, okay, creating strength does require some effort and some discomfort. But what I'd also never understood was that it was never supposed to be more than I could handle at a time, that I could be pushed gently and then dazzled by what a little pushing amounted to when accompanied by small, steady curiosity about what might come next. The secondary gift of all of this became the delight of self-discovery, reawakening all the parts of me I didn't even realize I had.

Lifting weights like I did might not be for everyone. But it led me to undergo a process of deprogramming and reawakening that could help anyone. And it does seem to help a lot of people—over the years of writing my column, I've heard from readers of all kinds who do not lift weights or identify as lifters. I'd hear from innumerable people who were staunchly opposed to working out in general, but also from runners, climbers, Pilates devotees, horseback riders, amateur circus performers. All of them wrote to me because despite their skepticism of lifting, they loved to read about this new, expansive perspective about bodies and food and exercise that lifting had given me. Still, many of them swore to me on God and life and love and their grannies in their graves that they would never actually try lifting weights. And yet, over the years, they trickled in, doing a squat here, a bench press there, joining a gym, finding a lifting buddy, getting their first big personal record (PR). None of us are setting world records. But then they would write to me again and say how overjoyed, how relieved they are that they finally gave lifting weights a try. If I know anything, it's that the emotional and physical journey of a body is long. But our bodies are also where we live, forever and always. However we go along, we all deserve to know ourselves a little better.

Finally, I think it's important to point out that though our culture has reduced basic care of our health to a luxury, it is a fundamental human right. The fact that everyone does not have equal access to health care is a choice enforced by people in power. Basic health—health that is not in decline because it is constantly infringed upon and nickeled-and-dimed away from us—is a right and a freedom we are owed. I enjoy a number of privileges that make it easier for me to take care of myself; they are the same privileges everyone deserves, and we deserve even more.

Part One

Only on the firm foundation of unyielding despair, can the soul's habitation henceforth be safely built.

—Bertrand Russell

Body, they blame you for all things and they seek in the body what does not live in the body.

—Ilya Kaminsky

1

Twelve Hundred Calories a Day

IT WAS THE KIND of cold that made every sound, even the snapping of twigs and crunching of the ground, deafening. I was wearing sweatpants and a full winter parka over a base layer I usually save for skiing. The headphones in my ears were buried under two hats. I'd signed up to run a half-marathon in Central Park at 6:30 a.m. in January, which now felt like a sign that things had gone horribly wrong. I had frightfully little understanding of how I had come to be in this place, in this situation—braving the worst weather that New York had to offer with the extremely dubious goal of running very far for an interminable amount of time and ending up where I'd begun.

I checked in at the race start, which would also be the race finish, in the dim light of the winter morning, the wind slicing through the mesh in my sneakers and freezing my already always-cold toes. As I milled around stiffly with my fellow runners like so many zombies, the dry, dusty snow sifted under our shoes, and the scene lightened from a dusky slate to a dull iron gray, revealing miles of rolling snowdrifts and bare trees under the looming buildings of Manhattan.

The race began, and I plodded around the enormous ring of the park track, carefully grabbing tiny cups of Gatorade from the little roadside stands in such a way that none would spill on my thick mittens. The air felt sharp to breathe and dry with salt from the road—a road that arced into a painfully long and subtle hill. It was enough of an incline to dramatically slow my pace but not enough for me to feel that any altitude would ever be gained—an insanity-making hill, a gaslighting hill. I ended at the start again in just over two hours. Afterward, I walked gingerly to a Le Pain Quotidien nearest to the race finish, and as my muscles stiffened, I ordered the not one, but two breakfasts I'd earned.

"Did you just run a race?" a man sitting with his wife at the next table asked, gesturing to the numbered bib I'd forgotten to take off.

"Yes, the Manhattan Half; it was just around the park," I said.

"Pretty cold out there!" he said. "My daughter runs, too—lots of races. I don't understand it, would never even try it. But you should be proud of yourself!"

I smiled weakly and thanked him as my breakfast was set down in front of me. I was starving from not having eaten anything before the race, but still I hesitated. I knew if I didn't eat, I'd barely be able to stand again, not just from tiredness but because my muscles would harden and cramp if I didn't refuel them with some of the calories I'd just lost. I wanted to, but I didn't want to, torn between hunger and guilt. Even the calories I'd "earned" I couldn't bring myself to eat. Even this reward, this prize awarded in service of these events taking place between 5 and 9 a.m. on a Sunday—a time forsaken by God himself—was refusing to justify and give shape to the assembly of choices that had led me here.

Still, I was emulating a type of person who I felt existed, real enough to touch: the runner who just sincerely loved running in all its forms. Her life arranged itself in an orderly way, a steady series of peaks and valleys. A determined mindset and positive attitude yielded consistent training in the face of adversities acute and chronic: energy, time, scheduling, weather, injuries. "Simply not feeling like it" was not in her vocabulary. This training yielded achievements, followed by the rewards of personal satisfaction and a large stack of pancakes. And then, in spite of the pancakes, she remained gracefully lithe, athletically slight. All was the result of her cheerful enthusiasm that sprang mysteriously, beguilingly, from within.

By the age of twenty-seven, I might have appeared like this to people who knew me or followed me on social media. I had the fancy running shoes, the time-and-distance running app screenshots, the photos of my bibs, sweaty selfies. All the pieces were there. But they were like demagnetized lumps of metal I kept pressing together, only for them to fall away from each other and lie inertly on the floor. Instead of feeling triumphant, desirable, hot, masterful, in control, I felt like a gray dishrag fighting to hold on to the edge of the sink lest I get washed down the drain.

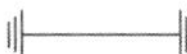

The great irony of it all was that I had always hated running. In high school, I'd participated in as many sports as I was able in hopes of burnishing my college application, and the worst part of every practice, bar none, was running for running's sake. Even running a mile was a unique injustice—the pain of drawing breath, the stomach cramps, the aching feet, the jouncing up and down at a pace I strained to keep steady despite feeling like I was fighting for oxygen with every step. After gritting through a long list of extracurriculars and APs, I found myself with a full ride to Columbia's engineering school. I planned to never think about sports again, let alone jog even a step for its own sake. I was an adult now, and no one could make me.

I did not anticipate that running would creep back into my life like an assassin, moving through the house silently closing doors and locking windows until it had me cornered (and there was, ironically, nowhere to run). Yet by midway through my junior year in college in 2008, I'd gained a solid twenty pounds. I felt ashamed of the person I saw in photos.

I'd been worrying I was fat since I was about twelve years old. In ninth grade, one of my biology lab partners flipped our textbook open to a chart of body weights and heights according to gender, next to a mathematical formula. Per the book, a healthy woman should weigh 100 pounds plus 5 pounds for every inch she measured above five feet. That means that a five-foot-two healthy woman should weigh 110 pounds; a five-foot-three woman 115 pounds, and so on. Christina had leaned over me to look at the table. "I'm five foot seven…one hundred and thirty-five pounds! God, I have some work to do, then," she'd said. I studied the chart: I was five foot six, so, I was supposed to weigh…not 137 pounds. My stomach sank. No one was going to let me know I was ten pounds overweight? I had to learn it at school in front of everyone? Who else had seen this chart and probably looked knowingly at my wobbling arms, my jiggling stomach, and guessed correctly that I was an entire house cat's worth of body weight astray of health? In mirrors, I began searching my body for the offending weight so I could monitor these areas closely.

By college, I was fully trained in the science of flaw spotting, well taught by the images of and commentary on female celebrities' bodies in TV and magazines. After I'd gained weight junior year, these reflexes kicked into high gear when I saw myself in photos or the mirror—Sagging waistline! Stomach rolls! Flabby arms that "wave back"! A too-round face and vanishing chin! I studied my body in the mirror, turning this way and that, longing to find a good angle. I decided it was time to try the 1,200-calorie diet.

I shrank all of my meals accordingly: toast for breakfast, soup for lunch, cereal for dinner. When I cut down, a few pounds quickly disappeared, but as soon as the diet began, I was longing for its end. I suddenly felt bombarded from all directions by all the foods I couldn't have—cookies, pancakes, bacon, burgers, fries, chocolate (except the one square per day approved by all doctors quoted in magazines). I saved a photo of Angelina Jolie as Lara Croft to my computer desktop to remind myself what I wanted to look like every time I thought of food. I saved a photo of Jessica Simpson wearing mom jeans and a wide gold belt, a photo that had led the media to refer to her as "Jumbo Jessica," to remind myself of what I didn't want to look like every time I thought of food. A few more pounds disappeared. And then...nothing. My weight loss slowed to a crawl.

I did the math: If 1 pound was equal to 3,500 calories, with an 800-calorie deficit subtracted from the standard-issue 2,000 calories recommended per day, I should be losing 6 pounds every month. Instead, after a couple of months, I hovered unsteadily around 145 pounds, losing a few before climbing back up again: 144 pounds, then 143, then 146. Then 144, then 142, then 145. I would double down and strive to eat barely anything, skipping meals back-to-back—142. I gave in and ate a regular meal—147. For eight months of grueling effort where just seeing a brownie could send me into a helpless loop of only thinking about brownies for the rest of the day, I had only about 9 pounds of weight loss to show for it. And that was just on one given day; I always risked the possibility of suddenly weighing more if I ate much of anything.

I was mystified. As straightforward as weight loss always sounded when everyone talked about it, my body did not seem to understand. *I* had to be the problem, some kind of anomalous, genetically deficient gargoyle that needed even more discipline than what normal people seemed to get by with.

There was nothing for it. I was going to have to work out.

2

Cardio

WHEN I BEGAN THIS self-improvement regime, I was in my junior year of college, and the summer was fast approaching. Though I always spent the break at home in upstate New York, where there were no ready bodies of water, I became possessed by the idea of being "bikini ready," in the unprecedented event someone whisked me away to an ocean or a lake. One night in my dorm, lying on my twin bed with my computer balanced on my stomach, I typed in a search for "calorie-burning activities." I'd had some exercise misfires before: a "core workout" from *Cosmopolitan* magazine, or twenty minutes trying to get my heart rate into the "fat-burning zone" on the elliptical at the campus gym. I was determined that this time it would stick.

Pretty quickly, I landed on a website that listed any activity's calorie output. Walking, 300 calories an hour. Lifting weights, 200 calories an hour. The idea of doing something as undignified as exercising for entire hours was unimaginable. But one of the highest calorie-burning bangs for the buck, at 600 calories per hour, was my old nemesis: running. Fifteen minutes of running would buy me 150 calories, or almost exactly three Oreos. Perhaps it should have said so in the first place.

I started by setting out for a run in the park near my dorm on the first warm spring day. My purposeful pace lasted all of sixty seconds before I had to slow to a walk, flushed and panting and out of breath. The pants and sweatshirt I was wearing were perfect for protecting me from the spring breeze but too hot for running. All the horrors were back: the pain of breathing, the mockery of how impossible it was to find a steady, sustainable pace. Once I regained my composure, I picked up the pace again, only to get winded after another forty seconds and slow to a walk. I thought of Jessica's stomach in her mom jeans; I thought of Angelina sprinting through the jungle. I hauled my body into a jog again.

As I threw myself at my little fifteen-minute running workouts over and over again, they became less difficult, if not less torturous. Over the next few years, I laddered up into running 5Ks, then 10Ks, and then half-marathons, taking out bigger and bigger cardio loans to buy myself more calories. I tore through Brooklyn and the Lower East Side, faster and faster and for longer and longer. My outfits streamlined from sweats on seventy-two-degree sunny days to shorts and T-shirts, even when it was cloudy and forty-eight degrees.

In fact, running started to become the only way I could generate heat; when I wasn't running, I was cold all the time. I continued to struggle with the breathing part, to draw and let go of breath at regular intervals, and I often felt like I couldn't breathe into anywhere below my ribs. But I just put up with it, panting shallowly mile after mile. Five years after I started running, I clocked a 7:18-per-mile pace in a 10K in 2013. That same year, I began to finish my half-marathons in under two hours. And most importantly, I was racking up hundreds of calories burned during every training run, which I could carefully, cautiously, occasionally spend on foods that I thought about constantly: a handful of chips, two cookies, tiny portions of candy.

As the runs got longer, I worked to ignore the fact that working out for more than about forty-five minutes would tip me into the realm of needing to refuel and rehydrate during the workout with sports drinks and energy gels, lest I "bonk"—become so depleted of energy that I'd induce extreme weakness, dizziness, nausea, the shakes, a pervading sense of doom, and even blackouts. Consuming calories during the workout would undercut the number of calories I'd burned to enjoy *after* the workout, so I resisted giving in as long as I could.

During my first nine-mile training run, I decided that I wasn't about to sabotage my hard calorie-burning work with eating any more than I needed to. I logged the whole thing with only a few stops at water fountains and then walked to a nearby Whole Foods. As I shopped, I felt my face getting hot and my breath getting short; the world seemed to be fading in and out. I fought my way through the checkout and collapsed into a chair in the dining area; I'd almost blacked out from not eating food, literally in the middle of a food store.

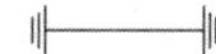

Why did how I look matter so much to me? The truth was that, in a certain way, it didn't. Or at least, I didn't want it to. Sports and, by extension, exercise were to me little more than a smoke screen of "well-roundedness" with a cynical purpose (college admission). What really mattered to me was my brain, my clever little thoughts, the books I read. These were also my best defense. What I knew could protect me: if a situation were to arise where someone asked the speed of light or why the caged bird sings or the right way to wash linen, I wouldn't have to flail, inviting scrutiny of what else might be inadequate about me. I collected information and thoughts and concepts in which to bury myself like so many giant feather duvets, obscuring and obfuscating everything about my physical existence that didn't involve my head.

I actually hated to have to think about how I looked. It was superficial to care, and self-centered to want attention for it. The idea of putting visible effort into any of it was abhorrent, and I was ashamed that I cared so much. But the idea of failing to clear what was presented as such a low bar—*Just lose some weight*—was even more so. There seemed to be few higher crimes, few ways of superseding and overshadowing all of the things I did and cared about, than "to be fat." To be fat was to undercut everything else I did, in a way that would grow larger as I grew larger. But if I could shrink, the reverse would happen: every effort would be magnified. So I dieted, and then I ran, and then I ran some more.

By the time I ran that Central Park half-marathon in January 2014 at the age of twenty-six, and then tried and failed to eat my breakfast afterward, I'd fought my way down to 138 pounds, my goal weight since I'd been nineteen years old. I'd expected after all this time to finally, at this point, be able to relax. Instead, I felt like a comic book superhero being wrenched apart by a tram full of children in one hand and the love of my life in the other.

Over the next couple of half-marathons, I started to get searing Achilles tendon pain anytime I ran more than three miles. I pushed through another four months of training and all the way through the Brooklyn Half, which wound from Greenpoint down to the beach boardwalk of Coney Island. My Achilles began stabbing at me once again around mile three and didn't let up for the next ten miles. As I crossed the finish line with a view of the whole Atlantic Ocean, I'd never felt more abandoned. I'd given running everything I had, getting lighter to get faster, spending mile after mile listening to pounding dubstep music that sounded like robots being tortured, to drive myself to shorter and shorter mile splits. I'd sweated, I'd panted, I'd nearly passed out. I'd even lied for it, lied like a dog for this terrible excuse of a hobby when even my own ever-weight-losing mother faintly expressed concern about my health. *I'm fine. I just love running*, I said. *It keeps me in shape. It gives you time to really think. Plus: the endorphins.* I was lying so hard I didn't even know I was lying, lying even to myself.

All I wanted was to not think quite so much about it all. I'd been promised happiness, self-satisfaction, self-confidence, and acceptance if I did the cardio, burned the calories, and followed the diet. I'd remained empty and given it all of the possible room to fill me up. But the more I ran, and the more I felt like the running should sustain my self-confidence and body acceptance, the more it felt like I was running to barely stay in the same place, to remain the same husk, trying to fill the moat of a sandcastle only for the water to steadily reabsorb into the ground. I felt hopeless and dejected about the scattered detritus of my relationships with food, exercise, and my body.

As I limped home that day after the Brooklyn Half, I felt deeply disappointed and dejected, and ready to give up. But I felt one small truth burning inside of me, which was that I'd been to the very center of the cardio, dieting, calorie-burning earth. I'd given it every chance to give me all the good feelings it promised, and they were nowhere.

I thought back to a post I'd seen on the internet a few months before whose promises had felt outrageous, to the point of being laughable. I hadn't been ready to believe them. Now I was finally desperate enough to give it a shot.

3

The Reddit Post

TRAWLING THE INTERNET WAS, for many years, my job. I worked as a reporter and then editor for a science-and-technology news website, and much of what I did was reporting on scientific research. But I got particular pats on the head from my superiors for digging up news about tech or video games from dim corners of online: forum posts, blogs, comments on blogs, comments in forum posts about blogs. Those were also my favorite stories to write, because they involved not just combing online, but rooting out the context, the implications, the reactions to the reactions. Deep internet digging is an instinct that the algorithms will never take from me. The Reddit post that changed everything, though, was one that found me.

It was 2013 when I came into my apartment late at night after meeting friends at a bar, wrestling with the caloric math of the beers I'd drunk, promising myself I wouldn't eat now that I was home. One of my cats was stuck on top of the kitchen cabinets, where he was always eager to jump up but too scared to climb down. With great effort, unstable from the drinks, I climbed up on the narrow counter to maneuver him off. I tossed him onto the couch, where I flopped down and opened my laptop to scroll for posts to write about for work the next day.

My usual news aggregator, Digg, popped up as my home page. I was scrolling down, down, down, when my eyes ran across the headline "What Happened to This Woman's Body When She Lifted Weights." It was an old Reddit post from 2011 that was making a second round some time after it had enjoyed an initial surge of virality. The thumbnail image showed two versions of a body, too miniature to betray any meaningful difference, but my sizing-up lasers were armed. My brain always hungered for new photos of women to pick apart, to find a fresh crop of flaws for which to flagellate my own body later. But also, the work of gathering information on which types of exercises to do and, even more importantly, which ones to mortally fear was never over. If this post was offering to explain the threat that lifting weights posed to someone like me, I was all ears.

I clicked through and skimmed the post, where a user named Montereyo had posted her six-month weight-lifting progress. She'd decided she wanted to get stronger (and give herself the chance at getting in the pants of her gym buddy, she said) by learning to lift weights. She briefly ran through her program: a workout three days a week, alternating two different sets of movements (squats or deadlifts, bench or overhead press, etc.). She would lift a particular weight until she could complete five sets of five reps at a time. At that point, in the next session, she would add five pounds, use it till she could complete five reps, and repeat. By the standards of what I understood "working out" to be, this was minimal. She stated proudly that she was now squatting 85 pounds, deadlifting 140 pounds (I didn't know what "deadlift" meant, but it sounded intimidating), and benching 75 pounds.

She'd been struggling to eat enough: "I had a pretty healthy diet and a good relationship with food, so it surprised me to discover how much diet-related bullshit I had internalized. For example: for a long time, if 2 pm rolled around and I realized I hadn't eaten anything yet that day, my first reaction would be, 'Gee, good for you!'" But she wrote that she was finally getting in the habit of eating more: "I know I should probably start tracking it so I have a better idea of what *exactly* I'm eating," she wrote in the comments. "I can say that I have 2-3 eggs and toast every morning for breakfast;

I try to get protein through extra fish/milk/cottage cheese in addition to what I would regularly be eating." Finally, at the end, she linked a small gallery of her "progress photos": front, back, side, and a superhero pose where she flexed her biceps to either side, naked except for some underwear and some artfully placed censor bars. "No, I don't do any cardio," she added to the post, after many inquiring comments.

I studied her photos through the fog of my own calorie-depleted state, clicking through shots from the front, the back, the side. She was slightly smaller. Her abs were more visible, her arms more toned. I felt a stab of jealousy. I looked from the photos back to the description of her workout and back at her photos again. What was going on?

I'd had a few lessons really drilled into me over the years, and one of them was that "lifting weights makes you bulky." Trainers and coaches shuddered and wagged their fingers and shook their heads at the very idea of women using weights to work out; there was simply no reason to do it, they said, unless your goal was to become a hulking, knuckle-dragging, no-necked gorilla with forearms like two ham hocks, legs like tree trunks, boulder shoulders, and a back like a bag of boa constrictors. *If your goal is fat loss, that "long, lean" look, stick to cardio to burn calories and lose body fat,* they said, *with some occasional Pilates and yoga to tone and lengthen.* And true, that was all I wanted. But I'd done the dieting—*Keep the calories low; eat small amounts of filling foods slowly; feel your hunger; deny your cravings.* I spent between six and eight hours a week running about twenty-five miles.

Aside from the calorie burning, I'd done the "toning" work. The fitness instructors of gym classes and magazine workouts, and now Instagram or YouTube video workouts, grinned out at me maniacally, asking if I could *feel the burn*; if I knew that *no pain meant no gain*; if I knew that *sweat was my fat crying.* I'd trusted their grins, their own ropey toned arms, their tans, their abs contouring their tiny waists. But the magic they assured me was taking place simply never came to pass; not only did my body seem to stubbornly remain itself, but I felt I could never step off the aggressive dieting-and-running merry-go-round, and worse, I only felt more discouraged about staying on as it spun faster and faster.

And all the while, here had been Montereyo, *not* following any of these instructions *and* doing the opposite in every single way: lifting weights, not working out that much, eating a lot. And she was not turning into the Incredible Hulk. She was achieving all of the results promised by the opposing side. She was standing straight and tall, her posture impeccable, despite the fact that she had done not even a second of barre or Yogilates. Not only was she achieving results, but she was actually having fun and feeling good about it, a place I'd longed to be yet never felt further from. How dare she. How *dare* she.

As I pored over Montereyo's post in my tiny apartment and wrestled with my simmering guilt over drinking beers, I was reminded somewhat of glowing testimonials I'd read in magazines as a teen, pieces meant to counterbalance all their content about the best fruits to eat for weight loss or the latest move to chisel your abs. The women in these pieces had found themselves through some new and unconventional form of exercise, and it had completely transformed their own bad relationships with their bodies: *I hated myself, I dieted all the time, I worked out too much and loved myself too little. Then one day, I decided to do everything differently; I found some new hobby [Olympic shot-putting / Muay Thai / volunteer fire rescue / recreational lion taming], and I realized that I needed to love myself more. I realized that being hot simply doesn't matter. And most importantly, with a little self-compassion, you can, too.*

These journeys were always presented as simple pivots, but to me they were an affront. The article might as well have reassured me that I, too, could walk on the moon if I just "loved myself more." Each day I faced an avalanche of instructions and admonishments about my appearance, all the potential pitfalls, all the wrong things to eat and do. And they had the audacity to stand there and say, "Actually, being attractive just doesn't matter"? What were they going to tell me "doesn't matter" next: Having shelter? Breathing air? I didn't even believe that hotter people were the "winners" of life, that being hot made someone a better or more worthy person. But I didn't get to decide what mattered to everyone else. And what mattered to everyone else, they seemed to yell from all directions, was appearances.

The photos that accompanied these articles were always of women proudly beaming, coated in sweat, post–some remarkable physical achievement, perhaps with their loving family or friends looking on. No makeup. No summer body. No coordinated outfit. While everyone else was out here grooming themselves and posing for the gods just to get a glimmer of approval, here was a woman proudly displaying her unvarnished self, spitting in the very face of composure and convention.

I hated and resented the self-satisfied "you'll understand someday" tone of these pieces. It was more than just the smugness; even if these stories challenged some of the values about the hard work of hotness, the framing still capitulated to the game. It picked not playing over not winning and tried to retcon that story into a success. It was like when people push you to do what they've done in order to validate their own choices, pulling people off the cliff we are all trying to scale, the cliff from which they'd decided to let go.

The most offensive part was the way these articles suggested that *their* lack of willpower was actually *my* mental damage, that my struggle to keep my head above the "basically attractive" water was something wrong with me personally, and they were proof. It enraged me, this "you'll find out what really matters" bullshit. I didn't create the cliff; I didn't even actively choose to start climbing the cliff. I was just here somehow, on the cliff. I was climbing the cliff because it's what you do on a cliff. Montereyo's post, at least, was not lecturing me while surrounded on both sides by juice cleanses and ab workouts.

But it wasn't just her post that grabbed me. The response to it had been overwhelming. People showered her with compliments on her strength progress and willingness to give strength training a shot in the first place. Not a few people complimented her progress photos.

"I don't lift to be hot," she replied. "I lift to be strong." I rolled my eyes. *Liar.*

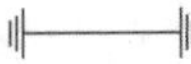

My unhappiness and desire to disappear had emerged in earnest when I got to college in 2005, and my dorm made a fast transition from HQ for my exciting yet fuzzy-focus adulthood to the best hiding place I'd ever known. I folded myself into my cinder block–lined room like an octopus. I had a computer. I had instant ramen. I had a little contraband slot toaster that was against fire code. Away from my family there was no one else to worry about, no one in my business, no inquiries to answer about why I wasn't where I was supposed to be, or why I just did what I did, or what I was going to do next. In a family of six, I'd always suffered for space, mental, emotional, and physical. Things only got worse when I turned eleven and we started moving houses almost yearly, meaning the renegotiation of that space was constant. I now cherished the isolation of my dorm room so much that I regularly fought the urge to go down the hall to pee. When people knocked, I did not answer.

I dodged every call from my parents, who had spent three years fighting in divorce court before I started high school. My older brother and then the younger moved in with my dad, while my sister and I stayed with my mom. At college, I watched their phone numbers pop up on my flip phone's display, and simply waited until the phone stopped ringing.

I was particularly befuddled by my dad's calls. In the year or so before leaving for college, my sister and I would visit him and my brothers on Sunday afternoons. He loved to play short-order cook and make us New York deli and restaurant food—tuna melts and tomato soup with dill sprinkled on top, pot roast, shrimp cocktail when there was a good football game on. He'd tell us about the new diet he was on—Atkins—for reasons that were unclear to us but perhaps for weight loss, maybe in anticipation of eventually dating again. We'd eat as he set in on a few beers, and my heart would sink as his eyes glazed over and his words began to mush together. I'd feel as if I were in a room with a wild animal pacing back and forth. I had to stay focused on not making any sudden movements that might activate it. I smiled and laughed at his jokes, casting around for any way to respond that would keep things on track.

One day while visiting home around Thanksgiving during my first fall semester, I ran into my dad in the parking lot of my mom's apartment complex as he was exchanging my younger siblings. My dad, at sixty-three years of age, scarcely ever picked up his pace above a brisk walk, so I was shocked when he practically ran over to hug me. I hadn't spoken to him in a couple of months. "Pick up a call from your dad once in a while," he said, clapping me on the shoulder a little too roughly to balance out his overly vulnerable desire for a hug, a sloppy gesture that reminded me of when he was drunk. "Okay, Dad," I said in my by-then-perfected teen pitch of detached exasperation.

I got back to the cocoon of my dorm room after the break, and he kept calling; I kept spectating the caller ID and held my breath after the ringing tone fell silent, as if some sort of retaliating gesture might burst through the phone. None ever would. I'd exhale.

One day, my older brother, Mac, chatted me on AIM. "Why aren't you answering Dad's calls?" he asked.

"I don't know," I said. I learned later that Mac had come home late at night and discovered our dad on the steps of their apartment, his face bloodied from a bar fight.

"You have to," he said. "You're killing him."

4

The Loss of Strength

SEVEN YEARS LATER, SOME things had changed: I was established in my own New York City apartment and had more of a social life and a job that made me feel like I was grown. Instead of isolating in my dorm room, I was out training for half-marathons, though I still tended to dodge calls from family.

But after the disappointing Brooklyn Half and the ongoing pain of running with an injured Achilles, I kept returning to this thread on Reddit. This woman's post, whether she meant it to happen or not, presented something different than I'd seen before. There were no exotic locales, no esoteric sports, and most importantly, the workout didn't sound like an avalanche of busywork bullshit; it sounded easy. It also didn't sound like something I would automatically be failing at if my abs did not emerge fully formed after ten days. Plus, she was eating. I had, quite frankly, never seen anyone speak of food in any proximity to exercise without framing it exclusively as a means for weight loss—as in, the less, the cleaner, the purer, the better.

It had been ingrained in me that to eat after a workout at all would be "wasting" the workout. For those who have never done the math at home, burning, say, 300 calories via exercise—about the equivalent of a piece of toast with peanut butter on it—is hard goddamn work. That's thirty minutes of running, or an hour of walking. What it takes most of an hour to burn, it takes about ninety seconds to eat again. This kind of math turned food into my mortal enemy.

But this Reddit post preached, if anything, the opposite of dieting. Montereyo said she was flagellating herself for occasionally accidentally skipping breakfast, not for eating it. If she didn't eat, that meant her muscles were deprived of important fuel that they needed. If they didn't get their fuel, *that* was wasting the workout.

Montereyo also had to make peace with resting. Her training program was only three days a week, leaving four days invisibly programmed for doing nothing at all. More work would burn more calories and overtax her muscles, throwing off the program's careful balance. I was reading this at the peak of #nodaysoff, when trainers like Jillian Michaels and Tony Horton were building cultish followings of millions of people off their insistence that fitness came only from annihilation of the self at the altar of "as many hours of exercise as humanly possible."

Finally, Montereyo's post was hard evidence that lifting weights, for a woman, was not unnecessarily excessive in terms of intensity or difficulty. It wasn't even risky or dangerous, not in terms of safety or in terms of threatening to make this woman balloon into a greased-up, stage-worthy body builder. She was a normal person, having a normal person's relationship with this activity that I'd previously understood to be reserved for macho gods and immortals, eating an amount of food that I'd previously understood to be reserved for people who had renounced the hotness battle I was locked in.

The element that really blew a hole through my belief system, though, was that Montereyo hadn't actually lost any weight. Not a pound. "I thought that lifting makes you gain muscle mass?" posted one commenter. "But it looks like you mostly lost fat by lifting? how does that happen? are you dieting too?"

"I am not dieting, as in, actively trying to lose weight," Montereyo responded. "I think I have gained muscle mass and lost fat—the number on the scale has stayed pretty much the same over the past 6 months." As I flipped through other parts of the same subreddit, I saw people discussing even more topics and techniques I'd never heard of before: bulking, cutting, cheat days, macros, hypertrophy, and body building (which seemed to be differentiated in some way from lifting weights in general).

The big problem, of course, was that this could all be fake, or at least overblown. In the land of exercise and dieting, it seemed nothing was ever as simple or straightforward as described on the tin. But as a journalist, I itched to know, always, if a story was too good to be true.

I went further down this rabbit hole, and soon I found hundreds of transformations on Reddit, sets of before-and-after photos of headless bodies along with increases in the amounts of weight they were lifting. Post after post showed leaner bodies, happier faces, and reported body weights that had barely changed. The process of "recomposition," the same process that Montereyo had done, had taken r/Fitness by storm. A million thoughts ran through my head. If all this were even remotely true, I had to tell… someone. But who would I tell? What would I say?

If there were such a thing as a "friend with whom you'd try a new diet together," I didn't have one. More to the point, I seemed to pick friends who tacitly agreed those kinds of subjects were shallow, or at least subjects of shame, to be chipped away at in darkness. Besides, conversations like that always felt to me like they could tip too easily into implied criticism. I'd never shared anything body-related with anyone, really, beyond the broadest strokes of running success.

Despite my best efforts, my most recent romantic relationship had just ended. He was handsome and sensitive and loved to teach me about photography; he had an eye for good light and took beautiful pictures of me and everything else. We bonded over wasting our precious youth on video games we fiercely loved. But we also fought often, conversations that began innocuously until they became hours of him lecturing, fretting, or imploring, and me crying but adamant not to give in, until the early hours of the morning.

As the relationship progressed, I began spending what felt like the majority of my time googling relationship advice, communication strategies, even possible mental health issues that might explain and steer us away from his high-strung, nihilistic, and despondent approach. I knew things weren't going well, that he was often unhappy, that he was controlling and jealous. Still, I figured all I had to do to save the 90 percent of the good in the relationship and eliminate the 10 percent of the bad was to dedicate myself to the question of how we were making that 10 percent go left.

In my endless relationship-advice research, which sometimes involved poring through forum posts of people recounting their own circular arguments with their significant others, I came across a book entitled *Why Does He Do That? Inside the Minds of Angry and Controlling Men*.

At the time, I was superstitiously careful not to make any waves or step out of line at my job. Despite my best efforts to have a more stable career, I'd ended up in media, and especially in the unstable economy, I was determined not to mess it up. Still, I was desperate enough for answers that I shirked that whole workday and read the entire book in one sitting. Eyes glued to the pages, my mind was blown over and over about the insidious dynamics of control, manipulation—however "unintentional"—and, a new-to-me term, "emotional abuse." All things that didn't have to be constant in order to be unacceptable, at any time, for any amount of time, regardless of anyone's "communication" or mental health. *Oh.*

I remembered one night the previous winter, when he'd arrived at my apartment so we could go to an industry holiday party I'd been invited to. I opened the door, and immediately he said, "Wow! You look amazing." As I gathered my coat, he took me in. Then a pause, then a smile, and then, "I've never seen you wear lipstick before."

"Yeah, I do sometimes. You know, red: holiday."

We made our way to the subway and stood on the platform, and he just kept looking at me, then looking away and shaking his head a little. "I've just never seen you wear lipstick before." I wasn't sure how to respond.

Women wear lipstick? Yes; I am a woman and do, in fact, own lipstick. "Why tonight?" he said.

Up to this point, I'd thought he was kind of into the lipstick, even if he was being a little teen-boyish about it. Now I wasn't so sure. On some level, it felt like the clock had started ticking: I needed to answer enough of his questions, well enough, that he wouldn't rule against me. I told him I'd already said it was a holiday thing.

"Yeah, but we've gone to other holiday things where you didn't wear lipstick."

I racked my brain for the other holiday parties we'd gone to—one at my friend Kelly's house; a bar gathering in the Lower East Side; a housewarming for my friend Sierra where he'd gotten upset that I didn't seem happy enough that he was there. That night we had gone many rounds: him saying he should just leave; me trying to convince him to stay, then relenting and saying he could go, which caused him to press me about why I "didn't care" that he left, until I got so frustrated at being unable to make myself understood that I ended up crying in a bedroom. Lipstick-less, of course. It seemed like so little was separating us from just having a good time, like we usually did, if I could just say or do the right thing.

What could I say that could save this holiday party, that would make sense of both the choice to wear lipstick tonight and the choice to not wear it the other nights, without either being evasive or having to explain myself at length? It was like a puzzle, where if I could just turn the pieces the right way, they'd click together. I rose to the challenge.

We boarded the train. "I thought I'd mix it up," I said.

"But why mix it up *tonight*?"

We continued batting the lipstick back and forth until we got off the train to walk the remaining blocks in the bone-clacking cold. I started to walk faster, trying to physically escape this argument, but he strode to keep up with me, maneuvering his feet so that he could walk and face me at the same time.

"Is it for someone?" he said.

"Who would it be for?"

"I don't know—it's your party. I don't know who's going to be there." I had no response and tried to walk still faster. "It must be for someone. Who is it?"

"No one! It's for me! It's not for anyone but me!" I yelled.

He stopped as I breezed past him. "You're mad. Maybe I should let you just go."

I stopped and looked at him. I knew from the experience at Sierra's party that what he wanted wasn't to part ways, or to be talked back into coming with me, but for both of us not to go. But he wouldn't say this directly and would only continue the argument until I landed on this "solution" myself. My stomach knotted at the choice between another endless argument and being cornered into not going to the party, so I chose a third option that felt nearly nihilistic. "Fine," I said, and turned to keep walking.

"Okay...well...bye!" he sputtered resentfully. He called out something else a few seconds later, but the distance and traffic prevented me from hearing it.

I went into the party, frustrated and disappointed in myself, ruminating and playing the argument over and over in my head. I felt confused and angry at him—why couldn't he just let the lipstick go? But I also felt guilty: I saw the lack of resolution as my own failure to adequately communicate why lipstick and the party mattered to me.

Months later, after reading this book, I was not so sure. I had been plagued by worse and worse self-doubt through the entire relationship, avoiding more and more choices and activities and people knowing it might spark an argument. But this new information sent me digging back through all our bewildering interactions, this new framework clicking piece after piece into place. Abusive relationships had, in my head, meant dramatic life-and-death situations worthy of Lifetime movies, not arguments over lipstick or whether to go to parties, for God's sake. Even with all of this new evidence, it felt like a leap of blind faith to actually end it. I spiraled some more for a few weeks and then finally broke up with him for good.

I told my mother the basics—that we had broken up—and she encouraged me to process my feelings through exercise by going for a run. "Maybe," I said, the idea curdling before me. I'd never told her about the deeper relationship problems; I knew better. It would have either sent her into an emotional panic where I'd find myself reassuring *her* that nothing was really wrong and I was fine, or she would've been skeptical of my perspective and taken the opposing side. She was the opposite of the right person to bounce all this lifting stuff off of.

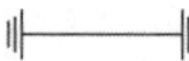

Whom I could confide in about this fitness discovery aside, I didn't even really know what I knew yet. All I'd done was struggle mightily with one approach and read about another one that seemed to have a nearly uncanny answer for every problem I'd ever had. And I barely believed it. If it were all true, if it were possible to do everything the opposite of what I'd been doing and not suffer, it would raise the question of why it was all so overlooked.

I was used to thinking of my body as having two components: "all the essential stuff no one can do anything about," like organs, skin, and bones; and "body fat, which it is our solemn obligation to eradicate from the face of the earth." But there is another component I'd scarcely thought about, which technically belongs in the first group: my muscles. I had always thought of my muscles as a basically immutable part of my body, like softer bones. I knew there was such a thing as "muscle loss," but that was for older people who had been confined to their beds by comas or grievous injury. To my mind, muscles sat there clinging to my skeleton serenely, waiting for me to lose enough body fat that they would finally get their day to shine lengthily and leanly from under my skin.

But this is not how it works, as I learned by falling headfirst into the science of bodies. Muscle is not just sitting there staunchly inside of us, and how much muscle we have is not an inherent and immutable biological quality that we are born with. Muscle has needs, and muscle can go away.

Muscle's biggest need is protein and the amino acids that make up protein. To sustain the amount of muscle we have, we need a certain amount of protein just for upkeep. How much depends on what we do—an Olympic weight-lifting athlete needs more protein to maintain their muscle than someone restricted to permanent bed rest. But we all have a number.

When we don't get enough protein, such as when we are aggressively dieting, our muscles can't take care of themselves. If sufficient protein isn't available, bodies have a ready solution for that: they can take existing muscle, chop it up into little bits, and feed it to the rest of the muscles that are wanting. In other words, muscles that aren't fed enough consume themselves and shrink away in the process.

This process can be pretty gradual, which means from the outside, it's almost unnoticeable, especially on the usual timescale of a crash diet. Muscle is also dense, as a tissue, so it takes up less space, pound for pound, than body fat. But that means losing it, not even that much by volume, has a big impact on body weight. Consequently, in the framework of "all body weight loss and lower scale weight is good," losing muscle is a "good" thing.

When I stopped giving my body not just the protein but also the calories it needed for such an extended period of time, while I was dieting and exercising and fighting to lose weight, it had pulled from my body's stores: yes, body fat, but also glycogen stored in my muscles to supplant the carbs I wasn't getting. Because my organs weren't getting the energy they needed by a long shot, they downregulated their functions. As this went on alongside the muscle loss, the balance in my hormones shifted, and my endocrine system began tipping out of whack; my dopamine cratered, while my cortisol, ghrelin, and leptin—stress and hunger hormones—shot through the roof. This would cause my cravings to kick into higher gear than ever, my body desperate to restore balance, but mostly to get its hands on any calories at all, especially the ones that could be delivered to my suffering organs—sugar, salt, carbs. The more I pushed, the more my body pushed back. The more I dieted, the worse and harder dieting got.

Muscle loss also has its own unique negative effects—sapped strength and energy, joint pain, moodiness. Since muscle is also the primary way our bodies use calories, less muscle also means lower metabolism. This means someone who diets and loses their muscle will have to fight progressively harder to maintain their lower body weight. Not only that, but when they inevitably regain the weight they lost, as most dieters do, and then attempt to lose the weight again, they will have less lean muscle mass and metabolic bandwidth to help them do it. This effect can repeat over and over for years and years, until you have an understandably very frustrated and physically depleted person who probably weighs the same amount as when they started dieting, but all the muscle that made their body function, that made dieting slightly easier, that is required for the "toned," lean look they might have been after is now gone.

During the months I was reading about recomposition, I would examine myself in the mirror in my underwear, studying all my body parts with fresh eyes. I dangled an arm; I shook a thigh; I contorted my midsection; I turned from the front to the side and back again. I'd always wondered when I'd finally manage to bear down hard enough that my body fat would dissolve away and reveal the toned muscles I should have from my monastic dedication. Now I was starting to see what was really going on: the muscle was gone. My body parts hung flat and deflated from my bones. I'd been digging for treasure and turning up nothing but dirt because the treasure had long since dissolved into the earth.

I had been, in effect, encouraged to diet aggressively with only a lower body weight in mind in order to always be losing weight and "taking care of my health." But the way these weight-loss-oriented diets undermined my body ensured not only that I would fail at the diet, but that I would subsequently regain weight that much more easily. Then I'd be compelled to throw myself back at that wall (harder each time), not knowing to blame anyone or anything except my own lack of will. It suddenly seemed awfully convenient that the central feature of most weight-loss diets—perfect circumstances for sustained muscle loss—would create a population that is ever-more dependent on more and more dieting in order to lose weight.

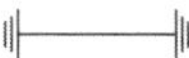

The lifting of the weights, at this point, I barely cared about. But the body composition aspect absolutely entranced me. All this time I'd thought of my body as just an amount of weight, and a thoroughly unreliable, unpredictable one at that. But this was because I hadn't engaged with what made up that weight, or how different kinds of weight might even affect the weight amounts themselves.

Everything I thought I knew was quickly crumbling: what calories did; where my muscle was, or how much of it I had; even what the point of exercise was. My unified theory of how these things fit together had never stuck. But there were dark matters and energies I had yet to discover that had pushed and pulled and dragged me around, manipulating the relationships between all of these things, impossible to see but whose effects were undeniable. To transcend them, I'd have to believe my own body first, which meant acknowledging it was even present and then, worst of all, listening to it. Well, ew, but okay—one step at a time.

5

The Scam

AS A KID, I climbed every tree and jungle gym I could find; I spent hours with my siblings throwing every kind of ball, both to and at each other. But as I got older, physical endeavors didn't feel as though they came as easily. When the opportunity to throw a ball came up, the reality fell shorter and shorter of my memory, the ball flopping out of my hand at smaller and smaller distances.

Much to my dismay, once I graduated from college, I found that being an adult involves an absurd amount of "picking stuff up and carrying it around." For instance, my meager budget demanded that I buy cat litter in bulk from the nearest store instead of paying to get it shipped to me. Since I couldn't afford a car in the city, I had to bodily carry home the largest box of cat litter I could find, which weighed 40 pounds. Each month I put off buying it as long as possible, letting the old litter dwindle down to only a smattering of its wettest crumbs, before going to the store to wrangle the brick of litter off a shelf and, with all my might, negotiate it onto the bottom rack of a shopping cart. This was the easy part.

Once the cat litter was paid for, I wrapped my soft little fingers around the biting plastic handle and began the shuffle of five long blocks back to my building. Every fifty steps or so, I paused for a break and to switch hands. Luckily, I lived on the second floor, which meant I had to drag the box up only about a dozen steps, bumping it hard on every one, praying it wouldn't burst open and spill all of my hard-won cat litter down the stairs.

Once inside my apartment, I'd pry open the spout and then begin the process of trying to pour the cat litter into the litter pan without also pouring it all over the floor. I'd prop it against the edge of the pan, which groaned while I tried to shift the weight of the litter up and over. At this point, usually the box would overcorrect, and the spout would face-plant into the bottom of the pan. With great effort, I'd try to pull the box out, and the litter would explode out, a deluge of tiny clay pebbles skittering across the floor, as the cats looked at me with, as usual, ungrateful disdain.

Lift with your legs and not your back, I'd always heard. But the cat litter seemed to be an object lesson in how impossible this little nugget of wisdom was in practice. All of my legs felt above the box, very not in a position to get near or under the thing in order to get it off the floor. As wrong as using my back supposedly was, I could at least contort it around whatever I was picking up and get some leverage going. The "right way" made no sense; the wrong way would eventually cause me grievous injury. Either my uncooperative body was preparing to eventually betray me, or there was something I fundamentally misunderstood about the basics of doing my dumb little chores.

One afternoon, in the spring of 2014, after a fresh and dark encounter with my nemesis, the box of cat litter, I sat back down on my couch with my computer. Even now, months later, Montereyo's post had never fully left my brain. My cupboard-scaling cat settled on the couch against my thigh and began cleaning himself so vigorously that he wobbled my leg back and forth. I opened more tabs that branched off of Montereyo's post. Soon, I was sitting in front of several tabs of beginner strength-training guides and had become the proud owner of the e-book version of *Starting Strength*, third edition.

Most workouts I'd encountered before online and in magazines were sunny and succinct tutorials led by lithe and smiling fitness models in coordinated outfits whose smiles reassured me that it would be *so* easy. Then they demonstrated a dozen or more complex movements that neatly divided the body into its unruly parts: chair dips for those flopping upper arms, side lunges for bulging inner thighs, planks to tone the core. All of this was gamely performed in photos or video, as the fitness models sweated not a drop, their hair perfectly coiffed. They harped relentlessly on the importance of "the core." One's "core," as described by Pilates instructors and fitness-studio advertisements, seemed to always mean the six-pack of abs on the front of one's stomach, visible (preferred) or not. Since high school, I'd attacked my core with all kinds of movements, from the exotic Russian twist to the astoundingly mundane sit-up or crunch (anywhere from 250 to 1,000 reps, as various celebrities including Britney Spears and Lindsay Lohan attested to doing). They never resulted in anything, except making it hurt to laugh or sit down the next day.

Starting Strength, by contrast, had no patience for all this; photo shoots and conventionally beautiful people cost money, so it was punctuated by black-and-white photos of normal people in a regular gym. Besides, all those little movements the fitness models were doing, it claimed, were time wasters. Bodies didn't need to be broken down into this or that muscle, worked individually, one after another, the book said. It made no more sense to try and exercise one muscle at a time than it did to try and walk one muscle at a time, or pick up a sock from the floor one muscle at a time.

What *Starting Strength* lacked in polish or flash it made up for with raw, unflinching, unsparing density. On the matter of "the core" interpreted by most trainers as "a part of the body that needs to be the entire focus of our workouts," the author was not impressed:

> Much is made of "core" strength, and fortunes have been made selling new ways to train the core muscles. A correct squat perfectly balances all the forces around the knees and the hips, using these muscles in exactly the way the

> skeletal biomechanics are designed for them to be used, over their full range of motion. The postural muscles of the lower back, the upper back, the abdominals and lateral trunk muscles, the costal (rib cage) muscles, and even the shoulders and arms are used isometrically. Their static contraction supports the trunk and transfers kinetic power from the primary force-generating muscle groups to the bar. The trunk muscles function as the transmission, while the hips and legs are the engine. Notice that the "core" of the body is at the center of the squat, that the muscles get smaller the farther away from the "core" they are, and that the squat trains them in exactly this priority. Balance is provided by the interaction of the postural muscles with the hips and legs, starting on the ground at the feet and proceeding up to the bar.

The more time I spent studying the program laid out in *Starting Strength*, the more I was struck by what a scam so much of "core" marketing now sounded like. We were being influenced to harp on and fret over our stomachs, this relatively tiny part of our bodies, because that was where so many of us naturally carried body fat, which left us vulnerable to being shamed into the penance of one billion crunches and planks. Meanwhile, the rest of our bodies were being neglected. But the core wasn't a standalone feature of the body; it fit into a bigger whole. It didn't need to be "targeted" relentlessly as the center of the body, because it *was* the center of the body; if the body was moving, using it was basically unavoidable.

Only a few pages in, the book dove into more complex physical and biological concepts: posterior chain, force production, eccentric and concentric movements. I picked my way slowly through the chapter over several days, jumping back repeatedly to the beginning, trying to remind myself of the big picture of how it all worked before digging back into the finer details.

There were over a hundred pages of text, black-and-white photos, and diagrams just on how to squat, a movement I'd previously understood to be no more complicated than "going down and up in a roughly-sitting-and-then-standing-up motion." It covered how to position feet, knees, butt, arms, and back, plus the relative angles of all of those things; how to move (up and down in a straight line), and how to troubleshoot various issues, like tipping forward, tipping backward, and the inability to reach "depth" (sink low enough in the squat that my hips traveled below the parallel top of my knees).

All of the pieces of the instructions stacked together to leave as little to interpretation about squatting as possible. Heels hip-width apart, toes pointed out about thirty degrees. Holding my back flat and straight (which was not the same as "upright" or "perpendicular to the floor"), I was meant to begin to bend my knees, tracking them in the direction of my toes as I also broke at the hips, lowering my butt as it migrated slowly out behind me, such that the tops of my shoulder blades moved in a straight line over the middle of my feet. I was to keep going down until the fold of my hips sank just below the tops of my knees—the point where I had reached "full depth"—and then reverse out of the movement until I was standing again. That was one squat.

A few days into this, after studying the photos in *Starting Strength* that modeled the squat, I stood up and cleared my desk chair from the bath mat–size floor area that doubled as my living room. I slowly lowered myself down, trying to hold all the cues in my brain: lowering my body while trying to get all my parts to move in the right directions, toward but also away from one another. My cat jumped off the couch and lay down between my feet directly beneath my butt, as if I'd just given birth to him, and began cleaning himself. My body stopped short as my hips caught, while my butt sank, rounding my lower back from flat into a curve. As soon as I felt myself tipping, I bailed and stood up. My knees squeaked in protest as I studied the book diagrams again.

A good squat would happen when my body's center of gravity was kept right in the middle, neither falling forward nor backward. I had to keep my weight over the middle section of my foot, neither on my toes so that my heels popped up off the ground, nor all the way in my heels. The whole point of the exercise was to stay centered and stable, even as I moved, even, eventually, under the pressure of weight. I had to rely on the feedback that was coming from within me and adjust how I supported myself accordingly.

The photos showed a sturdy man and woman compacted into a resting squat position. The man's palms were pressed together between his legs, elbows nestled on the inside of his knees, as if he were the benevolent deity of a new religion. I arranged my hands in front in the same pose and sank again; my knees obstinately sank toward each other, but with more of the weight of my arms in front, I eked out a few more inches of depth without tipping back. I could feel my tailbone tucking under like I was an embarrassed dog.

I suddenly remembered my all-girls high school chemistry teacher, who claimed to us once that boys could squat all the way down and keep their heels on the floor, while girls could not. "Prove it," we said. At the front of the class, he sank dutifully to the floor and crossed his arms over his knees, heels on the ground. He rested there as we all hopped out of our chairs and tried to imitate his movement; sure enough, every one of us toppled over like bowling pins. "See?" he said smugly.

And yet the images in the book defied him: one woman after another posed in the bottom of her squat, heels flat on the floor, often with multiple weights on her back. I grabbed a Swiffer from the corner of my room and laid it across my shoulders like the barbell the woman had in the photo and folded myself down again. I still felt that I wasn't getting quite low enough, but I was no longer being pulled off-balance in the bottom. I stood up again, then sank down again, this time resting in the bottom of the movement, studying the diagram and making tiny adjustments to my position—knees out more, butt extended out from under my torso as much as I could. My hips, hamstrings, and calves tingled with pain at the unfamiliar challenge of simply staying in position. I tried to push against the floor through my feet to stand up again and did so, wobbling a little on the midline axis. Just from these few squat attempts, my forehead was starting to pop beads of sweat, and the tiny room felt humid. I was beginning to see how even the few reps and sets of these movements might pose as much, or more, of a challenge as running six or seven miles at a time.

I flipped toward the back of the book, where the author brought all the lessons of the movements and muscles together into a single program. This beginner program was almost brutally minimalist: three movements per day, three sets per movement, five reps per set. For instance, one day consisted of squats, benches, and something called "power cleans," each for three sets of five reps. That meant an entire gym session consisted of only the following: A brief warm-up, then five squats followed by a minute of rest. Repeat twice. Five benches followed by a minute of rest. Repeat twice. Five cleans followed by a minute of rest. Repeat twice. Go home after a total of only forty-five reps. Perhaps most crucially, don't work out tomorrow. Then go back to the gym and do the same thing, except with squats, overhead press, and deadlifts.

A workout that was fewer than fifty reps in total? Benching, overhead pressing—I could figure those out. I'd seen them done out of the corner of my eye a thousand times before. But—I swallowed—the gym. I wouldn't just be doing these things in a little bubble of my own making—I had to do this in a gym, alongside the very types of guys who I was now watching in videos online as they confidently and rhythmically jangled and slammed their plates up and down in perfect deadlift form. I didn't look like them; I certainly couldn't lift that much weight, let alone lift it like the prima ballerina in the iron ballet.

Plus, the movements themselves were intimidating. Any time I'd bravely walked into a gym with the intent of doing a workout slightly more diverse than running, no matter how clear my purpose or detailed my workout, I'd always end up in the same place, dutifully studying the diagrams printed on the machines in the gym and letting them dictate the events. The machines always enveloped me welcomingly and gently pumped each muscle on their gliding tracks, rep by butter-smooth rep: a calf raise here, a tricep pushdown there, a machine-assisted crunch, a bicep curl. Usually, I found any more complexity in workouts intimidating.

But now, on the other hand, I was kind of entranced by the full-body efforts of the squat, bench, deadlift, overhead press. I'd heard of some of these movements, seen the equipment they happened on, and I'd even seen people do them, of course. The people who did them were always absolutely titanic, sweaty men in string tanks screaming for their lives as the stacks of iron plates rattled in their hands and on their backs while they tried to stand the weights up. The only way in which running had appealed to me was that I didn't have to interact with anyone in order to make it happen. Distressingly, it had to be done in public, but it had the benefit of also already being the way to secure safety and end any unwanted interaction: running away.

Now I was going to stick out like a squishy, brightly colored yoga mat trapped in a sea of metal and rubber and bullets of sweat and snarls of chest hair. I imagined myself again in the gym, watching myself in the mirror warily, trying to unfold my wayward joints in the right order, while a scary man stood by, getting redder and redder, his muscles swelling with rage until they busted out of his crop-top sweatshirt and gray sweatpants. I was standing in *his* spot, using *his* equipment, wasting *his* precious time, offending *his* hard-won sensibility. My heart contracted hard, and the feeling traveled up into my neck. If I wanted this for myself, there was no two ways about it—I would have to face the bros.

6

Hall of the Iron Kings

IT WASN'T LIKE I'D never been to a gym before. I'd gone to gyms like Planet Fitness here and there, chain locations that maintained an atmosphere not unlike a library. At Planet Fitness, I'd been surrounded by decorous, mostly white, mostly out-of-shape people like me, people who politely reracked their weights or gently pumped at the pristine workout machines. The equipment was so little used it barely needed maintaining, but was nonetheless dutifully wiped down on the half hour, every half hour, by attendants in matching T-shirts. These kinds of chains prided themselves on providing their patrons with a clean, orderly, and quiet environment, with safe, new equipment and ample lighting. These chains were trying to distinguish themselves from places like Richie's Gym in Bushwick.

For all the two years I'd been living in that apartment, Richie's had been just around the block, no more than a two-minute walk. From what I could tell from walking by, Richie's was a grimy independent gym, with barely comprehensible signage and metal grates covering the windows. Now, based on meticulous online research and much enhancing of grainy photos, I saw that Richie's had the free weights I needed: barbells, racks, and plates galore (unlike Planet Fitness–type chains, which didn't provide this equipment because it made too much scary noise). And compared to the fancier New York gym chains—your Crunches, your Equinoxes—whose prices stretched into the stratosphere, or cheaper chains that hoodwinked you into membership contracts that would follow you to your grave, Richie's cost only five dollars for a day pass or twenty-five dollars for one month's membership, no commitment required. I had not expected to find such a deal anywhere in all of New York City, let alone a block from my building. Despite being terrified of setting foot in this place, I was also clinically incapable of passing up such a bargain. With a deep breath, in May 2014 I stepped through its doors, my body armored in multiple layers of clothing, and asked to sign up.

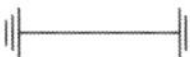

Richie's was lit like a warehouse, minus more than a few bulbs. The front of the room was crowded with cardio equipment and contained a handful of elderly people and young women pedaling quietly on the recumbent bikes or elliptical machines. They were watching TVs anchored to the wall, each one dysfunctional in a unique way: half static, garbled captions, stuck on one channel. But the cardio-doers' backs were to the rest of the gym, where most of the activity was.

The remainder of the gym's floor was wall to wall with every type of machine I could possibly imagine, a jumble of benches, racks, handles, pulleys, plates. The tops of the machines were coated with an inch of dust, while the usable parts of every piece of equipment carried years of visible wear: cracked vinyl seats, white cotton stuffing and poly foam flowing out of seams. The white paint on the metal piping of the machines was nicked and chipped not just at the corners but up and down their entire length. The 45-pound barbells were all bent in a curve from having hundreds of pounds loaded onto their ends, and the plastic-covered dumbbells were split and cracked from being dropped over and over again. Plates were haphazardly stacked out of order on every available peg, and whatever was left over was piled on the little floor space that remained. Above the walls of mirrors were spray-painted decals paying homage to gym-going legends: Franco Columbu, Lou Ferrigno, and of course, Arnold Schwarzenegger.

To get from one end of the gym to the other, patrons had to squeeze along small channels of a labyrinth walled by metal, vinyl, and sweaty, pulsing muscles, stepping lightly and nimbly to avoid tripping over the end of a 120-pound dumbbell or rolling an ankle on a large iron plate stacked on top of a small one.

The staff was blasting the latest rap, hip-hop, and R & B hits, from Pusha T to Cardi B, loud enough to drown out all but the rowdiest men and plates hitting the floor with a ground-shaking bang. The more crowded it was, the louder the music seemed to get. And Richie's was crowded, as I came to learn, almost all of the time. It was a zoo of bodies, most of them adorned with bulbous traps and wide, thick lats, droplets of sweat shaking from every direction, glistening where they landed in spots on the rubber-mat floor. A firehouse was around the corner, and its staff frequented Richie's, their bright-yellow equipment bags scattered across the floor and nestled in the nooks of the machines and benches.

As I took in the scene from the entryway, one man in jeans and a do-rag leapt onto the pull-up handles of the cable cross nine feet in the air to perform a muscle-up over the top, then a headstand, then headstand push-ups, his work boots reaching for the black peeling paint of the ceiling. More men leaned against the mirrors, curling 80-pound dumbbells, with pained expressions and beads of sweat popping out of their foreheads as their workout partners screamed at them to keep pumping out reps. An audience gathered around one very skilled and strong bencher as he set up for a 500-pound attempt, all of them yelling at full volume over the blasting music.

I hesitated near the front desk, feeling like if I stepped too far into the gym, I'd be swept up in its river-rapid current. The secure little bubble of my apartment felt very close and also a million miles away.

While most of my gym experience was with Planet Fitness–type places, I'd passed by enough weight rooms in bigger gyms to know they would inevitably be filled with big, intimidating men. I'd rarely dipped so much as a toe in these rooms but had heard enough about them that I felt certain of what to expect—staring, leering, hectoring, big-dogging; unwelcome commentary and even more unwelcoming attitudes; possibly unwanted touching or even grabbing. Men who wouldn't shut up; men who wouldn't leave you alone. I'd waged an entire mental war with the people I expected to encounter in this gym long before I even set foot in it.

So by the time I was actually standing on the shores of the teeming sea that was Richie's, my nerve endings were afire, coiled and waiting to lash out at the first man who dared address or approach me. At least that's how I felt. But as much as I would have liked to think I'd karate-chop the carotid artery of anyone who threatened me, I was far more likely to collapse into "reasonable and accommodating woman who politely laughs and smiles even if you are currently robbing her blind." Waves of apprehension flowed from knowing I'd quail and run for the hills at even the slightest challenge in this alien environment where I couldn't belong less.

Still, as yet, no one so much as batted an eye in my direction. They were too busy negotiating their equipment or bartering for the use of someone else's, doing reps, swapping seats to work in, changing plates for one another, balletically maneuvering around each other and toward and away from the room-length dumbbell racks. I might as well have been a speck of dust settled on top of the pec flye machine.

I'd memorized the workout I needed to do on that first day: squats, benches, and rows, for three sets of five reps each. These were the big "compound" movements from the *Starting Strength* book—all "push" or "pull" movements that used almost all of my body's muscles at once, teaching the systems to work better and better in concert with each other. No targeting, no isolating.

Squats, for instance, were a lower-body "push" that resembled standing up again from any height. Benching was a "push" that brought together delts, pecs, biceps, triceps, lats, and a bunch of tinier muscles into one smooth movement of extending my arms outward and away from my body. The overhead press—lifting a weight from in front of my face to over my head—was a vertical upper-body "push." There was the horizontal upper-body "pull" of the row, or the vertical "pull" of the pull-up. And deadlifts, the movement that sounded and looked the most intimidating of the bunch, were a lower-body "pull," most closely resembling picking something up from the floor.

They all complemented one another, and doing each one would help make the others easier. I didn't need to fuss over each individual muscle, one at a time, when I could use them all together, the way they were made to be used. The strength-training program would teach all of my muscles, disjointed and disconnected after many years of mostly sitting when I wasn't running as fast as I could, to come alive again and talk to one another. The workout never prescribed more than three sets per movement, and never more than five reps. Too many reps, too many sets, too many movements would interfere with the strength-building process. Doing no more than five reps at a time, with a weight heavy enough that I could basically *only* do five reps at a time, the *Starting Strength* text promised, would work my muscles in a particular way that couldn't be replicated by doing a lot more reps.

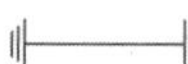

Arriving at Richie's, I had a clear idea of which dumbbells I wanted to try and use—the 10s first, followed by the 15s if the 10s felt too easy. But the dumbbell rack was virtually empty, nearly every piece in use or cast aside on the floor. I could see the squat racks off to one side, crowded with people, and the benches in the center of the room, also crowded with people, though one was open. I decided it wouldn't hurt to try benching first.

I slid onto the bench under the empty barbell and pushed it up and out of the rack. Already my arms shook unsteadily. The book had assumed the 45-pound barbell would be the starting place for its readers, so I thought it'd be worth a try. Now I was realizing this was a staggering mistake. I held it aloft, unsure what to do now; I'd look like a fool if I just put it back and walked away. Cowed by my hubris, I attempted a rep, lowering the barbell toward my chest, but it plummeted so quickly and uncontrollably I immediately gave everything I had to throw it into reverse to stop it from landing hard on my sternum. I felt my face growing red as I tried to force it away from me. The barbell swayed lazily and drunkenly in my hands, its ascent rapidly slowing down. I began to panic; this was among the stupidest things I'd ever done.

Just as the barbell's ascent slowed to a complete stop, a sure precursor to stapling me to the bench, two small, sturdy, tanned hands swooped in and grabbed it on either side of my face, yanking it up and back into the rack. My arms still hung in the air as I lay there, stunned. A smiling, upside-down doughy face with wire-frame glasses peered over me, framed by thinning, curly gray hair. I sat up and faced him, a rotund, olive-skinned man of indeterminable age. Though he wasn't aesthetically lean like the firefighters yelling at each other, his muscles moved visibly under his skin, which was exposed because he was wearing an open-armed ringer tank top, like an old-timey circus performer.

A grin split his face in two. "You lift-a *heavy* weight," he said. He seemed to be missing a few teeth that made his speech tough to understand, especially above the pounding music. He also had a thick accent I couldn't place—Greek, maybe. I pulled out one of my earbuds that had been part of my carefully planned strategy to discourage anyone from interacting with me. "What?" I said.

"If you ever want, I help you. Dimitrios," he said, pointing to himself. "Two fingers," he said, holding out his two pointers like finger guns and making a lifting motion. He was indicating a cherished bro custom I'd only seen parodied in movies, when one bro spotted another bro as he benched. If the weight on the last rep became too heavy and the benching bro looked likely to fail, the spotting bro would take his two index fingers and place them under the barbell, adding a seemingly small amount of support to help the benching bro drive through the last rep. As the spotting bro did this, it was customary to say, "Two fingers, bro, two fingers; I'm not even helping you—this is all you, bro," to preserve the benching bro's sense of accomplishment. Dimitrios was offering to spot me and help if I started to fail a rep, as if I were his benching-bro equal.

I nodded and smiled politely. "Okay, that's nice. Thank you," I said. "Casey." I pointed to myself, unable to let the introduction hang but also eager to move through this interaction; I was determined to keep any interloper at arm's length and wasn't about to make Dimitrios an exception, no matter how gregariously he offered to bro down. But if Dimitrios noticed how tense I was, he didn't care. "Two fingers," he said, holding them out again, "any time. You let me know." He ambled away, back to where he'd made camp in a squat rack arrayed with his full-size Igloo cooler and a beat-up rolling suitcase. There was a barbell set out on the safety arms with eight 45-pound plates loaded onto it, four on each side. He grabbed it and unracked it and proceeded to do rep after rep of shrugs, heaving his shoulders up to his ears as the hundreds of pounds dangled in his arms.

I'd been at the gym for less than ten minutes, and already, I'd done virtually everything I'd wanted to avoid—interacted with someone, made a fool of myself. But I was still alive.

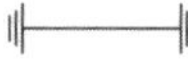

For years, I had hated how self-conscious I felt in these situations and how standoffish it caused me to be. So often, simply being out in the world with others caused me to feel uncomfortable. It was a double bind: I dreaded what I might bring upon myself by neglecting to be warm or accommodating enough, even as I knew the risks of being too warm or too accommodating. It was enough to make me want to write off the impossible game of all interactions, whether it was with strangers or friends or family. But I felt as threatened by isolating myself as I did by interacting.

When I had arrived at my first semester of college and I drank up the isolation like it was a spring flood in a desert, I'd continued to not pick up calls from my dad despite his requests, despite my brother's assertion that it was hurting him. At the end of my first college semester in December,

I traveled back to Albany and picked up shifts at Best Buy to cover their influx of holiday traffic.

In the middle of one of these shifts, my flip phone began vibrating in my front pocket nonstop. It was against the rules to use our phones on shift, so I ignored it. Then the corded phone at my register started ringing. My older brother, who also worked at Best Buy and knew how to manipulate the store's phone system, had patched himself through, right to my cash register.

"Why aren't you answering your phone?" he asked.

"I'm working," I said, feeling this was obvious from the way I had just picked up his call on a phone built into a Best Buy cash register.

"Can you take a break and go to the back? I have to tell you something."

I walked back to the break-room area and called him from my cell phone. "What's going on?" I said, irritated at all the to-do with phones by someone who was well aware of my emotional ineptitude with phones.

"Dad had a heart attack," he said. Everything in my body froze, suspended in bullet time. I waited for the follow-up: *But he's okay, this is where he is, here is where I am, here's what you do next.*

It didn't come. "He's dead," my brother said. Bullet time ended, and I felt slammed from the back as if by the seat of a bad roller coaster, carrying me implacably forward in the exact moment that I realized I would give anything to go back.

I went into the bathroom and locked myself in a stall and screamed, beating the walls and doors with my fists. Up until that moment, every existential threat we had experienced as a family had ultimately dissipated back toward the mean: my mom got in a car accident and lost half of her blood but received a transfusion in time and lived; my sister, too little to swim well, fell in a lake but made her way back to the shore; my dad had always made it home. The finality of this event—that I'd never even considered anticipating—pulled me under the surface.

I was hyperventilating, and I staggered against the wall over the toilet. But the wall remained infuriatingly indifferent to the seismic blow I was receiving from the linearity of time, the unfixableness, the impossibility of okayness, the realization that the net that had always caught me was no longer there and I was uncontrollably and unendingly falling.

A woman knocked on the door of my stall. "Are you okay?"

"Yes," I said between sobs; somewhere in the distance of my mind, I was incredulous at the commitment to appearances.

"Do you want me to get someone?"

Who? "No."

"Are you sure?"

"Yes."

She drifted away. I remained paralyzed in the stall for I have no idea how long, resisting any of the logical steps that might come next. They would only serve to turn this surreal moment into factual reality: leaving the room, telling anyone in charge that my dad was dead, that I couldn't finish my shift, getting in my car, driving away because I couldn't finish my shift because my dad was dead. I stayed in the stall as long as I could, futilely trying to protect my dad from being even more concretely dead.

I felt stinging regret over my revenge withdrawal, an action I didn't even understand and was now wild with desperation to go back and change. Our relationship could not have been irredeemable; there had to have been things that could be said and done to make it better. But during the time I had become so intent on avoiding it, unable to decide if I was doing the right or wrong thing, asserting a sudden incomprehensible-even-to-me blockade, the clock had run out.

7

Functional Movement

IN ALL MY YEARS of being alive, and then even in all my years of running focused on distance and time and caloric output, I'd never thought much about how my mind or body worked. They worked *enough*—less than I wanted them to and in a way that always frustrated and despaired me—and rarely seemed substantially moved by any intervention from me. Regardless of how I felt, even with my all-consuming efforts to lose weight via hours and hours of exercise and my strenuous, unrelenting resolve to not eat things, my body didn't seem drastically changed. If my body wanted to get fatter, or weaker, it appeared like that was barely any of my brain's business.

But perhaps the mistake had been treating myself as these discrete misbehaving little parcels to be herded and scolded and punished like schoolchildren. It certainly was convenient for the people marketing all of these body-part workouts that the more individual body parts there were to criticize, the more insecurities I had to tend to. In contrast, learning to use all of my muscles together, in functional motions instead of tiny muscle movements, was the point of strength training. In fact, rather than try to use each muscle individually in my upper body, like machines had taught me—delts, pecs, biceps, triceps—I could train them all together with one single smooth motion.

Take, for instance, the shoulders. When we think of shoulders in terms of muscle, most of us probably think of our delts, the bulbous caps whose size and shapeliness protrude from tank tops. In fact, shoulders are connected to our necks by the trapezius, which runs down the back of the neck and extends along the spine on each side, helping to stabilize the spine relative to shoulder movements. The front of the trapezius connects to the deltoid, the rounded upper-outer part of our shoulders, which can extend arms up and away from the body. Nested under these delts are the beginnings of the pectorals, which flow toward the center of the body within the chest, connecting at the middle, and which can pull arms and shoulders across the body and back again. Nested under that are the attachment points of biceps at the front and the triceps at the back, which connect the top of the upper-arm bone, the humerus, to the ulna and radius bones of the forearm. Biceps pull the forearm up toward the shoulder, while triceps extend it away again.

To move an arm in any one of these motions deliberately using only one muscle at a time, we have to be doing a pretty specific type of movement. In fact, the motions are so specific that I have a hard time thinking of an occasion I'd move one arm any of these separate ways, except in a specific type of workout, usually using a very specific type of weight-lifting machine built with the purpose of working that one individual muscle. But to move an arm in any of a dozen different normal everyday tasks—waving to someone, picking up a bag, opening or closing blinds—would combine some or all of these motions and, by extent, the muscles that perform them.

For instance, one of the fundamental motions of the upper body is to "push" things away from us, or ourselves away from them: getting cat litter into a litter pan, getting up off the ground. Pushing moving boxes into a truck, pushing heavy doors closed. There is not any single muscle that controls this motion. Instead, it goes like this: First, the muscles are loaded with force. To understand what this looks like, take your hands and hold them out, palms toward you, fingers pointed toward one another. Now slide your fingers so they are alternately interlaced with one another, until the tips of your fingers hit the nooks of your other hand. This entwined arrangement is the starting position of relaxed fibers. Now slide your hands away from each other, until the fingertips are all adjacent to one another. This is what a lengthened muscle looks like when it's loaded with weight, all pulled apart and stretched. Now slide your fingers together again; that is what happens when a muscle contracts to lift and snaps its fibers back together to shorten itself again and produce force.

To feel this process in your actual muscles, take one hand and hold it straight out in front of you, palm facing forward, like you are telling someone, "Hold it right there." Keeping your palm flat, draw your hand back toward your shoulder until your shoulder starts to roll backward and your elbow is tucked at a diagonal angle to your body. In this position, your pectoral muscle on the front and top of your chest is stretched, like a bow drawn back by an arrow. The stretching of the muscle matters because, like the drawn bow string, that gives it room and power to snap back into shape. To get even more granular, the snap of the muscles occurs when neurons fire among the fibers, triggering them to re-interlace with one another to contract the muscle, slinging the joint or limb in question with force. To experience this, now, with speed, press your hand back outward and extend forward from deep within your shoulder. That contracted your pec but also your anterior delts on the front of your shoulder, your triceps on the back of your upper arm, and a bunch of smaller muscles that either help stabilize your freely moving arm or act as antagonists to the action, pacing and controlling the motion, lengthening as the primary muscles are contracting, and vice versa.

These compound movements do make each motion more complex, since they involve more muscles and joints working together. But that complexity means the whole is greater than the sum of its parts. Having absorbed this, it made perfect sense to me; I didn't know why no one had ever explained lifting to me like this before.

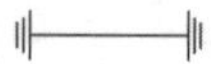

Starting Strength pushed using "heavy" weights to perform all the reps, but not "heavy" as in "several hundred pounds," which would be heavy for anyone on Earth. "Heavy," I learned, had to be defined relative to each person, their current ability, and the task they were doing. If I picked up two 10-pound dumbbells and squatted five reps with them and nearly couldn't do another rep, that was "heavy" for me that day.

And per the "training" aspect of things, "heavy" would be a slowly moving target that I would chase. If I could lift two 10-pound dumbbells today, even if that was all I could lift today, I would pick up two 15-pound dumbbells and be able to squat them the next session (theoretically, at least). I wouldn't get stronger any faster than that, but equally importantly, I *would* get that much stronger, in a matter of two days. Theoretically, at least.

I found this somewhat hard to believe, that strength building could be this straightforward and systematic, particularly for someone like me, who had not previously been recognized for her gifts in strength. I imagined there were people in the world who did get stronger, but I'd always assumed it was via arcane and complex training methods that would only work for those whose genes contained the secret strength-talent sauce. I would not have guessed it was something just any schmo could roll up to the weight room of the gym and make happen, because, well, if it were, why did so few people ever seem to be doing it?

8

Going Heavy

AFTER MY FIRST VISIT to Richie's, I decided that the long barbells were not for me yet, especially if I wanted to work out in peace. Within the next couple of days, I gathered the nerve to reenter its doors and start my first botched workout over. I moved through the crowd to the dumbbell rack, scouted around the floor, and finally collected a set of 10s. I took them to stand in a spot that I hoped didn't already belong to anyone and was in no one's way in the far corner of the room, at the very end of the dumbbell rack.

I hefted the two dumbbells up onto my shoulders and attempted my squats. After a set of five, I put the dumbbells on the floor and looked nervously around; now I was supposed to rest for a full minute or so.

Though the motion of the gym seemed constant, as I looked around, I could see a few other people resting, too, staring softly off into space or gazing idly around, their distant expressions suggesting that their most recent set had left them too spent to form any real thoughts. I did my next two sets the same way. In between, I toggled around on my phone, unused to so much dead time in a workout. Being any kind of semiserious runner involved long sessions of uninterrupted activity, where the entire point was not to stop. Now I was stopping every thirty seconds, for an entire minute. The rationale was that, because I was now doing more intense exercise, my cells were relying on their ability to produce bursts of energy, snapping off pieces of the chemical chain of adenosine triphosphate (ATP)—my body's main energy source—to create hot, crackly fuel. As I recovered between sets, my muscle fibers would rebuild the ATP chains using stored-up carbs, getting the chains ready to have their bonds broken again, freeing up that hot, fast energy. The resting between sets was essential to the whole program; if I didn't do it, my body wouldn't have the chemical bonds ready to snap. Part of me felt deeply emotionally uncomfortable during the rests, but I soon also became somewhat delighted for "just sitting there" to be technically a part of working out. From squats, I moved on to bench, this time with a nonthreatening 5-pound set of dumbbells.

I eyed some of the unused machines. I recognized the leg press, which was still loaded with what looked like a thousand pounds on either of its pegs from some meathead's sets. Beyond that, the twisting and gyrating bodies and metal swam before me. How was it that everyone else was seemingly going so hard, sweating bullets and rotating from machine to bench to floor, while I was only doing my dinky little three sets of five with barely any weight? I'd been thrilled with the prospect of this process being simpler than I'd expected. But watching the body builders and lifters and firefighters and bros expertly flowing through their complex workouts filled me with doubt all over again. Even if I was, very theoretically speaking, as welcome and entitled to a membership as anyone else that walked through the door, I was comparatively just an unsteady, unsure wisp bundled in layers like I was heading into a snowstorm. I'd never felt so small, which, by all accounts, should have delighted me. Even that, I couldn't enjoy.

The structure of my lifting sets, even, had been tough to wrap my mind around. How could something as simple as the numbers of reps make so much difference? Why would five reps at a time trigger the almighty "body recomposition," but twenty reps would be essentially cardio, just like running?

The information I was missing had to do with how bodies react to different types of activity. I'd always understood "strength" workouts to be (a) anything that wasn't cardio or yoga, especially if it involved anything that looked like a dumbbell or gym machine, and (b) a matter of doing lots and lots of reps (when you do a single crunch, that's one rep). More reps burned more calories, which caused more weight loss, or so went the theory of most of their sources. I'd never really thought at all about why these workouts were the way they were, and I'd never really imagined how they could be different.

Cardio and other less-intense forms of movement—Pilates, yoga, barre, any movement we can perform for multiple minutes at a time for many reps—activate our "slow twitch" fibers, also known as type I. These fibers are efficient at managing the energy we have stored up, and they are what carry us across very long distances with extremely repetitive, relatively light movements (hunting, gathering, migrations, and so on). If we are performing a movement we can do over and over again, we're not doing something that is difficult for our bodies. But "using up energy slowly" is exactly what these fibers are good at; they are meant to be slowly exhausted, not intensely challenged. (That's where the fast-twitch "type II" muscle fibers come in.)

This is why, when I'd done workouts that were sets of twenty or more reps, I didn't seem to notice much difference in either my strength or my ability; if anything changed, it was that I could do whatever the motion was for slightly longer than before. Strength training by lifting heavy weights, by contrast, was designed to challenge my body in a different way. And the difference was intensity.

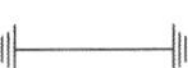

For this next part, bear with me, because to explain how cardio works versus strength training, we're going to dip into the world of plant maintenance. (Nothing works exactly like a human body, which is part of why it's so difficult to explain, but we never stop trying.) Let's say your body could be compared to a flowering, fruiting plant. Each day, the plant endures the trials and tribulations of being outside—wind, rain, snow, too much or too little sun. The stems and leaves make the little repairs necessary to keep growing, but the overall shape of the plant is leggy. Its energy is spread out over many small blooms, which weigh down the branches and keep them from getting as much light as they should. The fruits are small. The plant has worked and persisted through this time, but its ability to make fruit has been limited by its shape and size, which have been more or less static.

Now let's say before the blooming phase starts, you come in and do some light trimming of the plant, snipping off the tops and some extraneous branches, pulling up the smaller shoots to give the stronger ones more room and resources to grow. You've done some damage overall, but that's okay, because in time, the plant will repair itself, and now the lower branches will grow thicker and stronger. The blooms will come in larger and more robust. The fruits will be bigger, sweeter, and juicier.

This is something like what lifting weights does to our bodies. The damage caused by strength training does literally shred muscles, creating tiny tears as their fibers are pulled and lengthened by weights—like our interlocked fingers sliding away from one another until only the fingertips touch—then contracting with enough force to pull the fibers back in alignment again. But these tiny ruptures, this damage, create room and opportunity for more, better, and stronger muscle tissue to be built. In fact, this rupturing process sends the body into a repairing cycle, and it takes about two days for muscles to fully recover from this type of training (one of the reasons that I wasn't supposed to work out more than a few days per week).

Because the damage is overall pretty modest, muscle grows slowly for most people. A few pounds in several months would be a lot. (The total difference in even some of the most extreme before-and-after photos is only between twenty and forty pounds of muscle.) Because muscle is difficult to build, according to the testimonies of Montereyo and others, there was no reason to worry about giant muscles suddenly showing up overnight. The difficulty of the tearing-and-rebuilding process would be why I would lose some body fat simultaneously as I built muscle. But this body-recomposition process of losing fat and gaining muscle would also require food.

Taking care of a body and making sure it has enough fuel to live, let alone to grow back from the warped state it got into by eating too little, looks very different from "dieting for weight loss." Unlike weight-loss dieting, where eating too little is always good, eating too little while trying to build muscles can sink the whole project. It is possible to work out correctly and yet eat too little and have no recomposing sparks fly. In order for bodies to rebuild, they first need protein.

The US Food and Drug Administration has a recommended dietary allowance (RDA) of about 0.36 grams per pound of body weight per day. For a 150-pound person, this would be about 54 grams of protein. But newer research shows this figure may be flawed, and that our basic protein need just to prevent malnutrition in sedentary adults is about 20 percent more—65 grams for that same 150-pound person. For people who do any amount of physical activity, it's higher still—40 to 120 percent more than the RDA figure, or 76 to 119 grams.

People who are actively building muscle and strength, versus just "getting some exercise," need a significant amount of protein during this time, at least 0.8 grams of protein per pound of body weight (more than twice the RDA), and probably more like 1 gram of protein per pound of body weight (nearly three times the RDA). With that extra protein, bodies that have lost muscle can recover it again.

But to synthesize that protein into new muscle, bodies also need everything else other than protein that goes into a balanced diet to keep everything operating smoothly. Even if we think of a body as nothing but a factory for building muscle, the basic operations of muscle building—getting protein, breaking down that protein into amino acids, processing those amino acids into muscle fibers—can't happen without the complex web of macro- and micronutrients in all the other kinds of food to ensure that everything gets put to use properly. If protein in making muscle is the yeast in making bread, well—you need yeast, but if you have *only* yeast, you have no bread. You need flour and water, not to mention a baking vessel and an oven. Carbs provide the hot, crackly energy muscles need. And during this muscle-building process, with the right amount of food, bodies will also use up some of their fat. Which is technically, exactly one of the things that body fat is for.

I had believed that trying to eliminate fat at almost any cost was a perfectly healthy goal with no downsides. Yet despite its bad reputation in popular culture, body fat exists in harmony with all of the other types of mass clinging to our skeletons. Body fat is there, to some extent, to lose but also to gain. Fat is good for energy; it's good for insulating and protecting us and our organs and keeping our joints working smoothly. Fat was not the enemy, I was learning; fat was, in fact, one of the things that would make the whole muscle-building process work.

On Reddit, one recomposition post after another seemed to indicate that a body weight that didn't tick down, even while the person was working out or trying to eat in a specific way, was not itself a crime. This fact washed over the desert of my calorie-deprived brain like an ocean wave.

For my last exercise on that second visit to the gym, I tried rows. Bending over at the waist, I let the dumbbells dangle from my arms before pulling the weights up to either side of my upper body, upper arms at a forty-five-degree angle (or so I hoped, being unable to perceive myself). Three sets later, I was done. My second ever real-deal lifting workout, much more successful than the first, was rather suddenly over. I navigated around the bodies and benches and over the floor littered with plates and dumbbells to return my 10-pounders to the corner.

I thought back over my workout. Some of what I was supposed to be thinking about with lifting was how each rep and each set felt—too difficult? Too easy? Was I feeling it in the "right" or "wrong" muscles? Were other parts of my body hurting that shouldn't be? "Feel" was supposed to help dictate whether I needed to work on my form, or if I should add more weight. But I felt like I had no earthly clue what I felt. Part of the problem was that I was so focused on the goings-on of the gym itself I could barely think about what my body was doing. But the other part was that I had no sense of monitoring my body for "feel." What do you mean, "feel"? I could feel that it was there, I guess. I had a general sense it was moving. Beyond that, "feel" was a foreign concept to me. Feelings of the mind—sad, happy, distressed, forlorn, calm, angry—that was one thing (equally off-putting to me, but at least I understood the principle). Feelings of the body—before this basic lifting program, I didn't think anyone had ever even asked me about that before.

The main thing about lifting that had always worried me, other than "getting bulky," was that it seemed unnecessarily complex and even more intense. This emphasis on how it "felt" was a complicating element, one that bewildered me but that I thought I could safely ignore for now. I'd also always worried that lifting workouts had to be like what I saw the gym bros doing, cycling between tons of different movements for many reps. On this count, too, I was learning that this didn't have to be the case.

We often use the word "intense" interchangeably with "difficult," but here I mean it as "an activity that uses a lot of energy, in very few movements, over a short period of time." This, as opposed to "a lot of activity spread out over a lot of less-impactful movements over a long period of time." Neither type of activity is more difficult, per se. But lifting heavy weights is more intense, and that is why its impact is different, why it can be done in only a few reps of a few movements, especially for beginners like me. Intense movements like lifting heavy weights actually recruit all of our types of muscle fibers, the fast-twitch type II fibers as well as type I. And intensity was the key to why only a few heavy reps built strength.

Adding a little weight each time is what coaches call "overreach." If we do some training today, type II fibers can move fast and take an intense amount of activity (i.e., they can be damaged, just like the plant that we trimmed). After a workout, those fibers get rebuilt into more powerful versions of themselves, using the blocks of amino acids and nutrients and restocking with glycogen from carbs. By the time the next workout rolls around, the muscles have adapted to the amount of work we did the previous time, so they can take on a little more. And for beginners like me, it was supposed to happen that fast: If I was to squat 10 pounds that day, go home, eat all of my food, and rest enough, the next time I came back to squat, I would be able to squat 15 pounds, or even 20. The next time I came to bench, I'd use the 10-pound dumbbells and then the 12.5s next time, and then the 15s. This was how my wasted-from-too-much-dieting muscles would start to fill back in.

But the training, and subsequent increase in strength, wouldn't happen just within my muscles; it would happen between them, too. In practice with heavy weights, muscles don't even need to grow at first to get stronger; I would get stronger first from my body learning, rep by rep, to fire the muscles at the right time and fire them in sync with each other. The muscles that worked together to move my big joints—my hips, my shoulders—would, together, be able to move more weight than my smaller joints, like my wrists or ankles. Muscles that are trained to work together in sync are always stronger than any individually strong muscle working alone.

9

The Hunger

DURING MY YEARS OF multi-mile runs, I usually soaked through my shirt with perspiration, dripping as I boarded a train back home. But after my second weight-lifting session at the gym, I'd barely even broken a sweat. This left me deeply confused. The few reps of squats, bench, and rows felt like they had barely nudged my muscles awake. When I gathered my stuff from the little locker room to leave, I felt a twinge of worry.

And then as I walked out the door, there arose in me The Hunger.

One thing I can say for myself: I have experienced what it is to feel pretty hungry. I've been painfully, desperately hungry, so hungry that my stomach acid felt like it was boring a hole right through my guts—so hungry that I was weak in the knees, light-headed and dim-witted, unable to perceive any shapes and colors that were not loaves of bread. So when I tell you there was The Hunger, and I capitalize "The Hunger" in that way, you have to believe me when I say that The Hunger was different than any hunger I had felt before.

Previously, hunger had been defined by a lack, a neglect I could feel in the pit of my stomach. The Hunger, by contrast, felt like the blood in my veins had been replaced with lighter fluid and lit from inside with a match. From hip to toe and shoulder to fingertip, my limbs pounded the table and demanded sustenance like a tribe of Vikings returning from a holy naval war. The ocean of my body was a battlefield. The muscles had won, and they were demanding to celebrate their victory.

Instead of going home after my second, more-structured session, I looped around and into the nearest bodega. I ordered a bacon, egg, and cheese sandwich, and the cook behind the counter obliged, despite the fact that it was 8 p.m. I collected from the aisles a bag of hot Cheetos, an ice-cream Snickers, a bag of sour worms, and a strawberry-flavored protein shake. I paid for my bounty and carried it back to my apartment and straight into my bed, where I spread it out on top of the plastic bag, doused the sandwich in ketchup and hot sauce, and housed it all. I pulled out my phone and typed in all of the bits and pieces of the meal.

I had recently plugged my stats into an online "total daily energy expenditure" (TDEE) calculator. Based on my height, weight, sex, age, and activity level, the calculator would spit out the number of calories I should eat to maintain my bodyweight as I trained in the long term. I had set my activity level according to the amount of time I'd spend lifting each week (three times for about thirty to forty minutes), which was about half the amount of time I had spent on running. When I put the rest of my numbers in, my eyes bugged out at the results: the daily caloric goal was more than twice of what I used to allow myself.

Once I entered my bodega meal into my food-tracking app, I checked out the total: 50 grams of protein, 900 calories. Not terribly nutritious, but that was okay; post-workout was the time for the quick-digesting carbs to refuel my muscles so my energy didn't badly dip.

I lay back in the pillows and pulled up an episode of *The Good Wife*. I waited for the guilt and regret to wash over me: the junkiness of the food, the excess of carbs, the lack of "satiating" foods, how quickly I'd eaten instead of rolling every bite around in my mouth in order to "feel my fullness." But nothing came. My body absorbed the foods like a whirlpool. I was existentially nervous about this entire project, but I didn't feel terrible or overly full, the usual feelings that followed eating a lot. I felt like I'd met a clear need. And in that huge meal, I hadn't consumed all my calories for the day by half. I figured even if this "eating to support lifting" was all lies, if I overate by a few hundred calories a day, that should only equate to a few added pounds over the course of a month—a risk I decided to take in the name of the aesthetic results I hoped to finally get. I'd seemingly "gained a few pounds" overnight for no reason before; at least in this situation, I got to eat. Plus, I was supposed to be eating that much all over again tomorrow. I could hardly believe my luck.

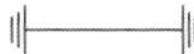

It's worth taking a moment to consider a particular kind of internal impulse about food—what we commonly refer to as cravings. Until relatively recently in human history, fat, salt, and carbs were difficult nutrients to come by, so our bodies evolved to instinctively crave them. They were also not usually completely isolated from all of the other nutrients; it was difficult to eat tons of carbs without getting a decent dose of fiber, because most of our carbs were whole grains, vegetables, and fruits. Now the single most available food is Doritos, a product that has had all the things resembling actual food distilled out of it.

It is a central tenet of weight-loss dieting practice that cravings are bottomless, and mastering cravings through denial and deprivation is simply part of being a grown adult. I believed this, too, from my perch of 1,200 calories a day and running five miles most days. If you eat, you gain weight. If you give in to cravings, you will eat a lot, which will mean you gain a lot of weight. That's just math. Or so I believed.

But cravings are not a bottomless human foible to conquer. They are rooted in our biology and can be related to whether we are eating enough—and enough of the right things—to sustain our livelihoods. Scientists saw this clearly once, but only when men's lives were at stake.

The Minnesota Starvation Experiment that took place in 1944 is one of the most famous trials ever, and its premise was simple: see what happens when a bunch of men don't eat enough and work out too much. The subjects ate only 1,500 calories per day and exercised intensively enough over twenty-four weeks to lose 25 percent of their body weight. While they did so, the men were closely monitored physically and psychologically. The findings were stark.

When bodies don't receive enough fuel, all of our biological systems get depressed. The men had reduced temperatures and blood pressure, and even their heart rates slowed. Our body's drive to restore functionality kicks in, which makes us want calories. Since we are efficient calorie burners, the quicker the calories and nutrients can be digested, the better. The body is so well-built to correct for starvation that people who are chronically over-dieted can even enter a "hypermetabolic" state when they go back to eating, where caloric math goes out the window and they can eat thousands of calories per day but barely gain any weight. (This probably explains more "models eating burgers who 'just can't seem to gain any weight'" than we realize.)

The symptoms of deprivation are not only physical. The starved men were depressed and struggled to manage their emotions. They even scored high for symptoms of hysteria, a typically female-exclusive medical diagnosis. Too much dieting, too much malnutrition, makes us deeply mentally unwell.

A prolonged state of deprivation also causes our brains to function differently in a number of ways: our senses become blunted, and we become hyperaware and rigid, even paranoid, about following rules (like, say, "never give in to cravings; you'll gain weight").

But we don't just crave amounts of food. We crave certain contents of food, too. Most of us may not have the biological attunement to distinguish between wanting potato chips and being in desperate need of, say, vitamin C. But there is evidence that shows that general malnutrition—that is to say, not lack of calories but lack of food quality and nutrient balance—contributes to cravings. This is a huge reason why we can down an entire can of Pringles and still be hungry. Part of it is how easily digestible the Pringles are, but another part is that our bodies' needs for all the complex parts of food—vitamins, minerals, fiber, protein, fats—are not being met. This means cravings can go another step further and create a vicious cycle, where malnutrition then feeds into an increase in addictive behaviors, even substance abuse.

In fact, cravings can even happen specifically as a result of too low of a protein intake. Research has found our cravings for savory foods and snacks can be a misread hunger cue for protein; one researcher went so far as to call these snacks "protein decoys." This was another reason that an actual, hard-number protein intake mark to hit was helpful to me: Following my hunger would not have led me there on my own.

I had not grown up feeling self-conscious of what I ate—until I got into my teen years and my body started changing. Countless times I would be in the kitchen preparing a snack when my mom would cross through, eyeing my stack of Pringles or Oreos on the kitchen counter.

"I see you've gained weight," she once said brightly, a smile frozen on her face. My mind began to race with answers: *So what? No I haven't. Thank you. It's actually this town that's gotten too small.* I was trying to find a way to respond that would not cause her to spiral into tears (because no one listened to her) or imply that I cared what she thought, inviting her to continue. I landed on a noncommittal "Okay."

From there, she kicked into high gear—she had spent the past few years studying for a master's degree in psychology, spurred by her own new experiences with therapy exploring her own history, as well as a deluge of self-help books—and she began diagnosing me, my eating habits, and my disinterest in discussing them with her as symptoms of anxiety, depression, trauma from the time my dad had gotten so out of control while drinking at home that the night had ended with him arrested, riding away in the back of a police car.

It was strange to me that she seized on this kind of moment, when there were many more mundane ones that barged around in my brain. One of my earliest memories was my dad, so angry and red in the face I was afraid he might kill me, hitting me with a wooden spoon for something I've never been able to remember—spilled glue, drawing on walls with markers, bringing dirt inside. But the worst moments were even quieter.

I thought often of the time we went out to dinner as a family (it had to be a special occasion to bring four kids) at a lakeside restaurant in the Adirondacks just north of where we lived. We kids returned from the sandy beach where we'd been seeing who could throw a rock the farthest into the water. I was only eight, but I knew how to count my dad's drinks by the liquid levels; I could tell he was on at least his second giant martini because the one in front of him was slightly fuller than the one he'd had when we'd run off. As I got closer, he turned and, after a few beats, smiled a faraway half smile at me. I knew well these too-slow motions and glassy, faded eyes, but I especially knew this smile; he never just smiled, except when he was drunk.

He swayed through dinner, eyelids drooping, eyes swimming, another martini half-empty in front of him. He normally had incredible comedic timing, but now when he spoke, the words and jokes dribbled out of his mouth like mush. Drinking like this usually subsumed my dad in a quiet, unstable calm, like an alligator gliding under the water. My mom was acting differently, but it was hard to say how because she was pretending to act the same. She shushed us when we made noises that would normally have activated our dad into an outburst, but he was barely aware of us.

When it came time to leave, my parents had an urgent, hushed conversation. We watched, waiting to be let into the van. "I can drive. I can drive," he said, taking the keys out and jingling them in his hand the way he did, fixing his gaze on the family van. My mom looked down and resigned herself to silence. I understood perfectly what was going on but also knew what the reactions would be to my inconvenient panic, so I stayed quiet, too.

The whole way home, I lay on the first row of seats in the back, eyes fixed on the rain streaming over the dark picture window opposite the sliding door. Each time the van swayed, changing lanes or speeding up, my heart beat faster. It was the twenty longest minutes of my life thus far.

Despite the abundance of these memories, I didn't want to add fuel to my mother's trips over my Pringles. I settled on glaring at her in silence and then took my chips up to my room, where I put them down and studied myself in the mirror, trying to find what it was that had made me a target in the first place.

10

Enough

WHEN I WAS GROWING up, to hear food discussed in popular culture, it was not at all apparent that someone who ate too little might be damaging their health. Foods were making you either lose weight or gain weight, and that was all. I never recognized my own hallmarks of disordered eating except in hindsight: heart rate fluctuations, low energy, constant feelings of cold, preoccupations with cravings, slow-growing hair, brittle nails.

I experienced every single one and never thought twice about them, because, troublingly, most of these symptoms are ascribed to "just being a woman in general." Women faint. Women are always cold. Women struggle adorably with basic physical tasks, like opening a heavy door, or throwing a ball, or carrying a suitcase. Women are always craving food they "shouldn't" eat. Women are meant to appear gracious in the face of deprivation, savor scraps, turn a simple biological imperative into an elaborate ritual of resistance.

In my high school health class, the teacher hammered home the signs of eating disorders: vomiting up meals, extreme restriction, extremely low body weight (unless the disorder was binging, and then, high body weight). We were visited by a speaker whose anorexia had been so severe that she had to wear special shoes because all the dieting had caused her to lose the fat pads in her feet, and that made it painful for her to walk. *Okay,* I thought, *as long as I still have the fat pads in my feet, I'm fine.*

Of course, I'd heard every health authority figure in my life—doctors, health class teachers—give the same vague instructions on what to eat for health, which was the same as "what to eat to lose weight and keep it off!": a "balanced diet," lots of fruits and vegetables. But the people who gave these incredibly vague instructions had the same credentials as Dr. Oz on *Oprah*, who said with complete confidence that African mango seeds would make me lose ten pounds. Shortcuts were, at minimum, presented as being on equal footing with doing things the "right" way.

Despite the fact that food and thoughts of my body ruled my waking life, and my health was meaningfully affected, I never received a diagnosis for an eating disorder. My weight was always in the healthy range (much to my dismay and despite my best efforts); my blood pressure at rest on the doctor's table presented as normal. I didn't even know to make anything of the dizziness or my gentle brownouts when I stood up (which were the result of dieting-induced sudden drops in blood pressure), or the unrelenting desire to eat a whole pan of brownies.

Only a small percentage of people would self-describe as having an eating disorder, and only a single-digit percent of people have a formal clinical eating disorder diagnosis drawn from the *DSM*—anorexia, bulimia, binge-eating disorder. But surveys about disordered behaviors highlight a much more pervasive pattern.

In 2008, right around the time I submitted myself to the 1,200-calorie diet, *SELF* magazine ran a survey of four thousand of its readers on their eating habits. It found that about 10 percent of them qualified as having a full-blown eating disorder of some kind, consistent with the rates found in the general population. But a whopping 65 percent of them exhibited disordered behaviors and thought patterns, some of which we think of as necessary in pursuit of health: trying to lose weight at an already-healthy weight; skipping meals; harboring concerns about what they ate or weighed that interfered with their happiness; becoming "extremely upset" if they gained even five pounds. "Although disordered eating doesn't have the lethal potential of anorexia or bulimia," stated the article on the survey, "it can wreck your emotional and physical health."

The survey had been supervised by the director of a research university's eating disorders program. But despite how revelatory it was, accessing a pervasive and damaging dynamic that was destroying women's senses of self and reality, it was not even advertised on the cover. The coverlines that were advertised instead: "304 tips to get summer sexy," "erase fat fast with the Self challenge," "slim & tone in just 30 minutes," "no-hunger tricks to crush cravings."

At the height of my disordered behavior, if I'd fought for it, I might have gotten a diagnosis of EDNOS—"eating disorder not otherwise specified." Today, I would get a diagnosis of OSFED—"other specified feeding or eating disorder." I would have fit perfectly into the OSFED criteria of what is now called "atypical" anorexia, which is more or less anorexia minus the low body weight. Despite the "atypical" designation, more than three times as many people have atypical anorexia versus "typical" anorexia.

On the other end of the spectrum from where I sat during my headiest dieting days was "intuitive eating," a trend to let one's food intake be guided by internal impulse alone. Intuitive eating was originally a concept derived from a book published in 1995 titled *Intuitive Eating: A Revolutionary Anti-Diet Approach* and written by two registered dietitians. Its thesis—that we could rely on our bodies to tell us what to eat, that there were no "bad" or "good" foods—caught on slowly at first and then began exploding. By the early 2010s, there was always a new person getting glowing press coverage for "just listening to her body."

It sounded great in theory; I'd never heard of it as a teen. It was targeted at helping people heal their relationships with their bodies when those relationships were previously built around food manipulation.

But coming from a history of deprivation, the instructions on how to rely on feelings and intuition felt, to me, ironically, like circular double-speak:

There are no good or bad foods, the intuitive-eating reasoning seemed to go.

Yes. Yes.

But when you listen to your body, you just won't want to eat certain foods, because if you do, they'll make you sick.

You mean the bad foods?

No, no—there are no bad *foods. Just…certain foods. But you should eat what* feels *good.*

Yes. Yes. Okay. Like ice cream and Doritos.

Yes. Or vegetables.

Huh?

Like roasted ones, with a sauce. Maybe you want some vegetables.

You mean Doritos and ice cream are bad?

No, they're fine; you just might not want them all the time.

But I do want them all the time.

Well, if you have them all the time, you'll feel bad.

I don't know if I'll feel bad; I think I might feel the best I've ever felt in my life.

You'll feel good at first. Then you'll feel bad. Then you won't want them all the time.

And I don't want to want them all the time?

Right.

So I…should have them all the time? So I won't want them all the time?

Yes. I mean no.

Because they're bad?

No—they're fine!

So I can have them all the time?

You can—but you won't want to.

So I should want vegetables.

You should want whatever you want.

Like Doritos?

Yes. Or some carrots.

And on, and on.

What is less discussed in the "intuitive eating" world is that even the intuitive eating bible, *Intuitive Eating*, recommends as its tenth and last step that adherents steer their way back to an existence of "gentle nutrition." "Gentle nutrition" is not an intuition free-for-all; it involves trying to eat according to our health needs but without turning the basic nutrition guidelines or numbers into a bludgeon of self-harm. This is, frankly, one of the most confusing parts of the book, with its heavy hinting at the need for rules after a book's worth of encouragement to throw the rules away—a final "by the way" that at least partially undermines everything that came before it. (Perhaps unsurprisingly, the "gentle nutrition" section does not get the same lip service in popular culture that the mystical, free-spirited "listen to your body" sections do.)

After all the years that had passed since I became deeply aware of what I ate in my teens, the prospect of listening to myself after decades of being buffeted about by PepsiCo, McDonald's, Nutrisystem commercials, and constant images of Britney Spears's midriff seemed like about as good of an idea as following a wild-eyed man in an overcoat into an alley. My "intuition" demanded both starvation and a one-pound plate of buttered noodles. Years and years of backward, upside-down situations had made its compass go completely haywire.

The problem I faced when I was willing to step back from dieting and give strength training a try was that I needed some way to figure out what to eat, today. Every eating framework I knew of either turned the whole experience into a highly ritualized form of torture (dieting) or left me to guess entirely for myself (intuitive eating). I couldn't just tune in to my intuition; stories of binging and confusion and guilt abounded for aspiring intuitive eaters. I was also coming off of years of, essentially, intuition-guided eating, to the extent it could apply in my little-calorie budget, and it had only done me wrong.

Once I finally began strength training, though, there was suddenly a different qualifier in place. The idea of trying to eat *enough*, a high minimum to support lifting, gave the compass a north again, a north that was beyond the reaches of my intuition and yet nearer in purpose than "my health" or any of the other usual directives—it put the experience of my body first. *Do you want to have a good day in the gym? Bring me these amounts of all these different foods.*

Eating to build up my strength provided me with some coherent and flexible rules. First, I needed to eat way more calories than I had ever before dared. Second, my protein intake had to be higher than I had ever imagined possible. Lastly, I could not cut corners in terms of the broad nutritional strokes: I needed fiber, but I also needed carbs and fats.

When I had plugged my stats into the "total daily energy expenditure" calculator, the calculator told me that my basal metabolic rate—the minimum number of calories I needed to sustain me—was 1,430. That meant for my entire adulthood while I was attempting to eat only 1,200 calories per day, I'd been trying to survive on even fewer than I'd need if I were in a deep coma. No wonder I'd been staggering through my life like the undead. I found I would need a whopping 2,250 calories just for recomposition.

Next, I needed to figure out my protein. When bodies are trying to build muscle, protein forms the building blocks: inside the body, protein gets broken down into amino acids, which reconstruct the broken-down muscle fibers. With enough amino acids (plus other nutrients to support the rebuilding process), the muscle fibers can be rebuilt better and stronger than last time.

Previously, I'd gauged my protein intake based on what food nutrition labels said. A couple of glasses of milk and I was basically there, I had figured. But the amount needed to gain my muscle back was way higher—at 0.8 to 1 gram per pound of body weight, I'd be shooting for 116 to 145 grams of protein every day.

What did that mean in foods? A palm-size serving of cooked chicken breast (about three ounces) has 25 grams of protein. Two eggs have about

15 grams. A cup of Greek yogurt has 23 grams. If I ate any one of those things in my old life, I would have considered it a "good" protein day. Now if I ate all three of them, I was barely halfway to my goal.

This was not to mention all the rest of my food. With about 600 calories a day going toward protein, I had a whopping 1,650 calories to expend between carbs and fats—again, more than I was accustomed to eating ever, period. The 15 grams of fiber per 1,000 calories I was eating would keep me on the right track as far as vegetables and fruits, but that still wouldn't take all of the calories to achieve.

While eating had always been too fraught with baggage to ever be really fun, with all these numbers swirling in my head, I now felt daunted by the task of wrangling and triangulating them all. It felt like I'd been trying to get through life using and reusing a plastic grocery bag, and now I'd just been handed a Louis Vuitton duffel. Not unrelated, I still felt unsure I could trust it—how could I just be handed a Louis Vuitton duffel? How could it be possible that I could have had a Louis Vuitton duffel all along, while all this time everyone had been saying I had no choice, that I was required to make do with the grocery bag? How could "eating almost nothing" and "eating a lot" be nearly equal experiences?

The journey from my literally birdlike diet to 145 grams of protein a day, though, was destined to take time. I played with my food-logging app and its vast, often error-ridden database, combing for high-protein foods and combining and recombining them into fantasy meals, like outfits in a closet. What did a double-patty versus single-patty cheeseburger contribute? If I got a Sweetgreen salad but doubled the chicken, where did I sit? It seemed that most average serving sizes were not going to get me there, and doubling the protein was always the key. I ordered two tubs of protein powder from the internet—one chocolate, one vanilla—and began adding it to my morning oatmeal, as well as drinking a protein shake after every workout.

I was surprised to learn that, in the grand scheme, many foods that I understood to be "protein foods"—peanut butter, Snickers bars, most nuts, cheese, milk, beans—actually had pretty pathetic protein bang for their calorie buck. If I made them the "protein" component of every meal, I'd end up far short of my goal. I still had plenty of room to eat those foods, but they would not satisfy my protein needs alone. Generally, I needed foods with a higher ratio of protein to calories than a glass of milk (about 10 grams per 110 calories). If the food had more protein than that for the calories it had, it was helping move the protein needle. I needed eggs, Greek yogurt, tempeh, tofu, and yes, chicken, beef, fish, pork.

This presented a little difficulty for the college-dorm-style fridge of my tiny apartment, which lacked a real freezer and was generally warm enough to hasten the spoilage time of most foods I put in there. Meat was gross to handle in a way that, say, a box of cereal was not. I also had no hood to my tiny stove, so if I wasn't careful, meat juices and grease spattered everywhere. This was a diet better suited to cavemen and cowboys than anyone packed into a city studio apartment, with her couch a mere three feet away from the kitchen setup. I trawled recipes for foods that wouldn't spray grease all over everything I owned: roast chicken, chili, meatloaf, coq au vin, casseroles, braises. I eventually got enough experience handling the meat that I didn't have to wash my hands twenty-four times per cooking session.

But once I started eating in earnest, the cravings I'd fought mightily like a Hydra with ever-sprouting heads miraculously vanished. Every couple of days, I stepped with trepidation on my bathroom scale, fearing the worst fate that could befall a woman who bravely ate more: gaining three, or even five, pounds. In the first week, my weight did jump around by that much, as I'd read it might. In the past, these weight fluctuations after workouts always unnerved me. But after about a month, it settled back to where it had been at the start. I was hooked.

It had never occurred to me that eating meals that consisted only of salads with no dressing or bowls of cereal or toast would have contributed to my dazzling food cravings. I didn't have to choose between "mastering" them or feeding them endlessly. They weren't bottomless. They were finite.

I felt my muscles before I could see them. Each day, as I practiced the lifts, the movements got easier. Instead of lurching over and bending at the waist to pick something up from the ground, suddenly I was squatting down without even noticing. Deftly pouring the cat litter was one thing, but it wasn't long before I could contort my body close to the giant 40-pound box of litter, wrapping myself around it between my spring-loaded legs, and pick it up without dragging on my lower back muscles.

My body was electrified with energy, and I was, of all things, for the first time I could remember, warm. That is to say, my fingers and toes didn't turn to ice while I sat at my desk in a seventy-four-degree room while wearing a long-sleeve shirt, sweatshirt, long pants, and a scarf. I didn't feel moved nearly to tears of relief by eighty-five-degree days. As spring shaded into summer in New York, I wore shorts and short sleeves and tank tops. When the occasional cold spring breeze blew over my bare arms, it didn't chill me to the bone. I could sit in the shade without it icing me over. My muscles were like those reusable heat packs made of rice, encasing my bones and organs, protecting me from the fluctuations of the outside world.

Each day I showed up to the gym with renewed energy, and each time I left, The Hunger came banging in in its zany, yet reliable way. I relished every new bountiful meal with all its different foods; along with all my protein, I ate avalanches of carbs and fats: Pop-Tarts and Oreos and bread with butter and grilled cheese sandwiches and milkshakes and french fries. All of the parts of myself that had been fighting each other, heart against brain against body against stomach, had beautifully Voltron'd into one functioning unit, united in the holy cause of getting strong as hell.

Part Two

The wound is the place where the light enters you.

—Rumi

You can only recover your appetite, and appetites, if you can allow yourself to be unknown to yourself.

—Adam Phillips

11

A Stadium of Lights

I KEPT SHOWING UP to the gym, and weeks of training began piling up. I never felt as if I was working very hard. Where I'd previously fretted over days I didn't work out due to weather or my schedule, only having to work out three days a week meant it was easy not to miss a day. And still, session after session, the weights I was lifting steadily increased, five pounds at a time. After several weeks, I was lifting dozens of pounds every which way. For some moves, I had graduated from dumbbells to barbells, even starting to add plates to barbells, stacking more and more on with each warm-up set.

I usually went to the gym during lunch when it was relatively empty, but occasionally, I still found myself having to lurk nervously near an occupied squat rack or bench setup, waiting for an opportune moment to interrupt the person using it and ask how many sets they had left. Some were terse bros, giant noise-canceling headphones clamped to their heads. But the fixtures who visited from the firehouse next door were much nicer. They would smile at me and gamely unload all the weights at the end of their sets to leave me with an empty bar that I could load up myself—a kind gesture, since I could barely maneuver one 45-pound plate myself, let alone the stacks and stacks that some gymgoers tended to leave (seemingly a tacit challenge to the next person who might approach: *You're not* man *enough to lift as much as me*). I was grateful that not only did most of the members not give me a hard time or operate in selfish ignorance of whoever else might be in the gym, but they seemed to genuinely care that I was as comfortable as they were. Dimitrios, too, continued to smile winningly as he passed by wherever I lifted, giving thumbs-ups and always offering to spot my bench. I would give him a tight-lipped nod, hiding how relieved I was to be welcomed.

Every few days, I stood in the mirror in my underwear, surveying my body for any of the promised recomposition changes. I studied my abs and arms for definition, my butt for lift and size. I knew it wasn't going to happen fast, and I was mostly so relieved to have a break from my previous exercise-and-diet life that I didn't mind. But still I waited impatiently, like a child for Santa Claus. And ever so slowly, more shadows started to develop across my body. My pants grew ever so slightly tighter in the legs and hips but fell away at the waist. The scale stayed the same, but my limbs, whose flesh previously hung solemnly from my bones, took on a 3-D effect. My muscles looked alive under my skin, like animals chasing each other under bedclothes.

Nowhere on my body changed more than my back. I'd always been hollow between my shoulder blades, thin skin stretched over the knuckles of my spine. But session upon session of rows and deadlifts called for locking in my back, holding it straight under more and more duress. Now the muscles that ran neck to waist began to pulse gently through, if I could get a glimpse of them—annoyingly, my back was the hardest part of my body to actually see. Holding up my phone to see my back's reflection, I tried to flex to make the muscles show, contorting and shifting my shoulders and arms and upper body around like a dancer interpreting a drugged ferret. But when I could get the positioning just right, the muscles sang. After a few months, they looked like a bag of...maybe not boa constrictors, but garter snakes, at least. I felt elated and astonished—there was a whole different person in there, in here, who had existed patiently, dormant under the surface.

To look at my body unflexed with clothes on, though, it appeared barely any different. At first, in my characteristically secretive and withdrawn way, I told no one about my new hobby. I knew what people thought about women who lifted weights, what they might assume my goals were—to become a hulking, tanned mass strapped into the teeniest little bikini on a body-building stage. The promise that had lured me in, though, had been that lifting weights would make me look different but, importantly, not vastly different. I tested this by keeping quiet and seeing if anyone did, in fact, notice.

People had long freely commented on my body, almost never with invitation—even friends complimented me when I showed up to a hang-out looking noticeably thinner. But true to the promises, no one seemed to experience even a shadow of concern that I was lifting weights, because they couldn't even remotely tell. So long as I didn't give anything away with a sudden feat of strength—tearing a phone book in half or picking up one end of a car—my new hobby was essentially a secret.

The rate at which people can gain muscle varies a little, depending on genetics and whether they are using performance-enhancing drugs like steroids. But assuming they are training consistently, eating well, and resting enough, the average woman is able to gain about a pound of muscle per month (if they are doing recomposition, they'd also then be losing a pound of fat a month). For men, the rate is about double—two pounds per month. This is only when they are untrained, and eventually the results taper off. After six months to a year, it becomes much harder to deliberately put on muscle. (Another point against the bulk fearmongers.)

But most of the transformation that was taking place in the early days was happening in my central nervous system. My body parts and the nerves that controlled them, formerly quiet and dark, began to fizz with electricity. At first it was just a few errant sparks, misfires of a long-dormant network. But every time I attempted to do a squat or a deadlift, I was swinging up the big handle on the breaker box of the haunted old theater that was my body. And when I did, the circuits flickered a little more brightly each time. The frayed wires started to heal, and the power started to flow a little more smoothly. New lights lit up, lights I didn't even know I had. The dark theater became a dim theater became an illuminated high school football field became a stadium concert tour's worth of lights. The pieces of me that barely worked previously, only dimly aware of one another, were learning to blaze brightly together. My shoulders lock, my back sets, my hips tense, and my feet drive the floor away, flooded with light.

As I returned to the gym again and again, my body a little more awake each time, I began to understand what was meant by trying to assess how each rep and each set and each movement "felt." With every new session, as I concentrated on the limbs and parts moving the weight, willing them to move, I could feel them speaking back to me. As the weights got heavier in my rows, the backs of my shoulders would ache with activity. Squats from which I could only get out of the bottom thanks to bouncing off the backs of my calves found new tension building in my hips. I started to develop a new wordless, physical vocabulary for all the new sensations and experiences I was having, cataloguing them like exotic birds in a jungle—too heavy and too light, but also the good versus better positioning of this limb to that one or relative to my torso, feet planted here versus there, weight held close versus too far away from myself.

I found that the mind-muscle connection, or the imagined dialogue sounding back from my muscles to my brain, wasn't just my imagination. Research from the last few years suggests that active muscle cells can send signals back to the brain, through the blood-brain barrier—in the form of proteins, in fact—that indicate they are working and may induce the creation of new neurons and new memories.

I wasn't even sure if I should tell anyone I was lifting, except that I was bursting with elation about the difference it had made in my life. I was eating and I was working out and I was resting, and all of these health-related tasks had made a near-immediate transition for me, from pits of despair to mountains of delight. Previously, all of my physical life had revolved around the dynamic of working and punishing myself for eventual rewards. But the way I went about it kept me doing more and more and more work for a reward that never came, only more punishment in its place. In lifting, the dynamic was reward, reward, reward: eat and rest to gear up for a gym session, have an amazing gym session because I ate and rested, go home to eat and rest to maximize the gym session, repeat and repeat and repeat.

I had gone so long without knowing about any of this stuff—and based on the way I heard virtually everyone talk about their bodies, based on the way so many people I knew longingly but guiltily turned down food or begrudgingly paid lip service to the idea of working out, other people didn't seem to know, either. Neither did I know that they would care, though. The thoughts that wanted to tumble out of my mouth bordered on religious zealotry: *You can lift more than you think—it's not even that many reps or sets. Then you go home and eat your macros—you know, like protein, carbs, and fat—and even if you can't hit depth in your squat, you can practice your form so there is no tipping or butt wink.*

Squatting had become my favorite of the lifts. It helped that Richie's squat racks came with built-in safety arms to catch the barbell, so I didn't have to worry about getting crushed by the bar in the unlikely event I suddenly collapsed. But I practiced my squat religiously, sinking down and camping out in the bottom to stretch my hips and calves and force my knees out over my toes. I was enamored of the idea of having a perfectly structural, solid squat. And every time I showed up to the gym, I was able to pick up more and more weight.

Despite the occasional struggles, I was possessed with how elementally different I felt. Physical acts that used to be, for me, some precarious form of lurching, like leaning sideways out of a chair to grab something without getting up, became suddenly effortless.

Near the end of my previous relationship, the doomed boyfriend had given me an orchid plant. When I finally accepted how bad the relationship was, I projected many of my bad feelings onto the orchid. I stopped watering it; I didn't put it anywhere it'd get light. Eventually, it dropped its flowers and became nothing but a couple of dull, dark-green leaves flopped over the surface of a tight, dry cube of moss and soil. As I grew, the orchid withered. This went on for about five months.

One day, I decided to try watering it and moved it closer to the window. After a few weeks, to my surprise, a tiny green nub appeared from deep inside the withered leaves, then another. New leaves sprouted. And when the weather turned brisk, the cold made the plant send a flowering spike snaking up into the air, and it popped open half a dozen new blossoms. It went on to bloom many, many times again.

In physics, there is a concept called quantum superposition. Textbooks explain it using the idea of a cat and a poison vial enclosed together in a box, unobservable. At some undeterminable time, the poison vial will break, and the cat will die. So if at any time you ask me, "Is the cat alive or dead?" the answer is that I don't know; the cat is in a superposition of "alive" *and* "dead." When you open the box and look at the cat, you "collapse" the superposition, because now you know. I'd thought the orchid was dead, when in fact, it was in a superposition. I'd thought that I was alive, and in fact, I was in a superposition. I hadn't known because I was too afraid to look. I'd been neglected for so long I'd thought the idea that I could grow was a joke. I had not realized how much I'd felt like an empty shell until I looked inside and found a person in there, barely alive but still breathing.

12

Stronger Than Men

A FEW MONTHS AFTER I'd started to lift, I showed up to a rooftop party thrown by a friend of a friend on the Lower East Side. People scampered between the crowded host's apartment on the fourth floor and the roof another two floors up. I was packed into the apartment, scrounging for a drink, when my friend Emma asked what I'd been up to lately. I thought about my experiment in secrecy and decided to end it right then and there. "I started lifting," I said.

"Like *weights*?"

"Yeah. At the gym."

A random woman in the jostle turned and caught my eye. "Don't you *love* to work out? I run every day to earn my scoop of Magnolia banana pudding."

"Um," I said.

My friend Dennis, who was over my shoulder, overheard the conversation. "Wait, wait, wait," he said. "Make a muscle." He didn't say anything about giant body-building muscles greased up under stage lights, though I could tell where his imagination went. I held back my *But wait, no, it's not like that* protest and simply turned to him. I held up my arm to one side, forearm flexed at an angle to firm up my bicep and try to make it pop. It barely responded. All that was visible was a gentle twinge underneath my skin. He wrapped his hand around my upper arm and squeezed. "Oh, come on," he said. "You got nothin'!"

"I know," I said, putting my arm back down. "But I really feel it. It's crazy how fast you get strong."

"Yeah?" said Dennis. "Arm-wrestle me."

"Come on."

"No, really!" By this time, the conversation had gotten the attention of a John and another, second John who were never far away enough from one another to be called just "John"—they were called by their last names, Sperry and Molinski. Sperry was always flirty with me, and I'd long had a bit of a crush on him, too. But I had always had a boyfriend, and anyway, he was rumored to have been semibetrothed to a girl who had recently moved to the city.

"Don't be chicken," Dennis said.

"I'm left-handed."

Dennis, flanked now by the two Johns, fixed me in a twinkling gaze before tossing his head. "It won't matter. Here—" He pushed through the mass of people to a table littered with party cups and swept some of them aside. He positioned himself on one side of the table, arm extended, elbow down, palm open. "C'mon."

I moved to the other side of the table, put my own elbow down, and grabbed his hand. Emma, who had followed us over, placed her hand over our gripped hands and counted down. "Three—

"Two—

"One—

"Go!"

Dennis's hand tightened around mine, and his wrist locked. I was no arm-wrestling expert, but I knew the cranking of the wrist was a hard move to come back from. I steeled my own wrist and began wrenching back against his arm. Sperry and Molinski whooped and screeched like wild monkeys. Our locked hands remained immobile for several seconds, betraying no bias toward my victory or his. And then, ever so slowly, they started to move. As Dennis's hand began to droop toward the table, his facial expression went from tense to straining, reddening with effort. But the redder he got, the faster the back of his hand descended toward the surface of the table. He managed to slow my progress down for just a moment, hovering one inch over the table before relenting and letting his hand finally drop. He jumped up, shaking his hand and making sounds of disgust. Sperry and Molinski booed, but their faces were lit up.

"Me, me," said Molinski. "Me, me, me, me." He slid into Dennis's spot across from me and offered his hand, which I grabbed. Emma again started us off, we locked hands, and before I knew it, Molinski's was descending to the table. By now, people were watching, and they cheered as he lost. As Molinski backed away, Sperry squared up, sure that he could do better than either Molinski or Dennis before him. I balked a little—already this was more than I had bargained for, in terms of making a particular kind of show in front of a crush. I hadn't even planned to disclose my secret identity as a weight lifter that night. And here I was, not only outing myself, but swept up in a public display of strength, having not prepared at all for a full-on free fall of how everyone perceived me.

But then I shrugged and took his hand, and Emma set us up, though Sperry's grip was already deathly tight on mine under Emma's hand. He gave me a challenging look, one eyebrow raised. When she released, the back of my hand started to dip gently toward the table. I steeled up and stopped its progress, unsure if I had it in me to recover. But I held firm, and after a few seconds, Sperry's tension began to fade, and our hands righted on the table before his hand began to fall toward the table, steadily, until it touched down. Sperry looked up, let go, and then took my hand again, this time to shake it as the gathered crowd cheered.

I could hardly believe my success at arm wrestling, even if it was only my three semi-wasted friends whom I'd beaten. But I'd wondered if I might be stronger than I looked—and even suspected that I might be—especially when it came to doing feats of strength over and over. I knew that, on average, the very strongest men could usually lift more weight than the very strongest women in a single go. But I'd also recently learned that this wasn't the only way of measuring strength.

I'd always heard that women tend to have more of those type I muscle fibers built for endurance tasks like running or doing thousands of crunches. Men, meanwhile, were purported to have more of the fast-twitch type II muscle fibers, used for raw-strength tasks like heaving boulders and carrying damsels to safety. In the fitness world, this was often flattened into "women should exercise like *this* (cardio, Pilates, gentle body-weight movements done for hundreds of reps) and men should exercise like *that* (lifting weights, hitting tires with mallets, picking up and carrying damsels to safety)." Once again, science was being used to make it seem like women have no place struggling and straining with heavy weights, exerting force, exhibiting strength.

But when I looked closer, these stereotypes were bunk. Women tend to have between 7 and 23 percent more type I muscle fibers than men. That's all. Not three times as many, or twice as many, or even 50 percent more—only a scant double digits percent more, in most people. If I have 100 jelly beans, and you have 7 percent more jelly beans than me, you would have 107 jelly beans. A random person looking at our two jars of jelly beans wouldn't even be able to tell the difference. This is not nearly enough of a difference to suggest that women ought to train night-and-day differently from men.

More to the point, these differences mean women are weaker than men *only* if we measure strength in one extremely specific way. Because of the diversity in muscle fibers, women's muscles tend to have a higher density of capillaries, and thus more blood flow, than men's do. This, combined with the impact of higher levels of estrogen and progesterone, means women tend to be more fatigue-resistant, allowing them to do more overall work than men's fibers before getting tired. Not only that, women recover more quickly, meaning they can get up and do more all over again, sooner. Is this (female) blend of muscle fibers, for certain definitions of work, superior to men's? Yes, actually, depending on how we define "strength."

Let's take an untrained woman of roughly the same height and starting weight of a similarly untrained man. Let both of them train hard, lifting heavy weights for ten years. At the end of that ten years, that woman can deadlift 400 pounds. The man can deadlift 600 pounds. These are not world-record-setting numbers but enough to make both of them nationally competitive. But usually, we'd say that the man is way stronger than the woman, because the way we usually define "strength" is "whoever can lift the most weight."

First, it would be ridiculous to say that a woman who can lift 400 pounds, or even 100 pounds, is not "strong" just because she may never be able to lift 600 pounds. To steer anyone away from lifting because they could "only" learn to lift a staggering 400 pounds instead of 600 pounds would be like telling someone they shouldn't go to math class because they might only become Neil Armstrong instead of Marie Curie.

And then: Sure, the man in this thought experiment can lift more absolute weight, once, in a single-rep attempt. This is how strength is defined in lifting competitions. But why? As we noted earlier, women tend to have a greater potential to do more heavy work on the same day and recover faster. Maybe the man can lift 600 pounds once, and he is wiped out for several days. But the woman is more likely to be able to lift 90 percent of her max, 360 pounds, for *five* reps in one go. In lifting, we would calculate the total "tonnage" of these reps as 5 × 360, or 1,800 pounds. The same man may only be able to lift 90 percent of his max for three reps, for 3 × 540 = 1,620 pounds in tonnage. If the gold standard of strength performance were total tonnage, and not one-rep maxes, it's very likely that women would be topping the charts over men on a regular basis.

Not only that, but women are more likely to be able to do five reps at that weight all over again the day after tomorrow, thanks to their superior recovery. The man, meanwhile, needs more days to lie on his fainting couch, waiting until his inferior muscles, with less blood flow and less fiber diversity, can rally back to fighting form. What if the hardest task were not doing a difficult thing once and then having to lie down, but being able to do it over and over again, on more days of the week, week in and week out?

But for a subtle shift in how we define our terms and how we set priorities in strength-training goals, women are, in fact, better suited and more genetically predisposed to strength train and work with heavy weights. It doesn't wipe women out as much. They can do more reps, in less time, on more days of the week. Perhaps men should leave the scary weights that tire them out so much to women, who can handle it.

After the arm wrestling that night at the party, we gathered our drinks and climbed the rest of the stairs to the roof. It was directly adjacent to the open structure of a neighboring building under construction, so close that people were climbing directly into and within it. Apart from the hanging lights in the half-complete building next door, the roof was dark. I looked over the edge to the street, which was relatively peaceful, given how late it was. A halal cart was the only animated part of the scene, its lights changing from blue to red to green.

As I looked on, Sperry grabbed my hand and pulled me around a corner to a less-populated section of the roof. He brought a bottle of Johnnie Walker Blue out from behind his back. "I stole this from Molinski's room," he said, unscrewing the top and holding it out to me.

I took the bottle, eyeing him, and took a swig before handing it back. He took a swig, too. "You're a badass," I said drily.

He took another swig without breaking eye contact. Then, looking down and back up, he said, "Make out with me."

"No."

"Come on."

"I have a boyfriend." Technically, I was lying, but I knew it didn't matter, because—

"Well, I have a girlfriend."

I took the bottle from him and took another swig. The moment hung there as I weighed whether this would be embracing someone who actually returned my interest or just courting pain through recklessness. The call did not feel easy.

I handed it back. "I'm not drunk enough for that," I said, and turned to walk away.

He held up the bottle of whiskey. "That's what I got this for!"

"I have to go now," I called back, smiling, swinging back around the corner to the rest of the party.

13

Deadlifts

WHILE SQUATS CLICKED FOR me pretty quickly, my body refused to make any sense of deadlifts. Deadlifts were the closest analog to "picking stuff up off the floor with your legs, not your back," a process that had mystified me long before my struggles with the cat litter. But even after a few months, I wasn't yet able to do a true deadlift.

Setting up for a deadlift required positioning my body around the barbell resting on the floor. According to my book, this was as follows: feet halfway under the barbell, shins leaning forward to just touch the barbell, torso bent from the hips over the barbell so shoulder blades were positioned over top of it. In order to get in that position, I'd need a 45-pound barbell with one 45-pound plate on each end set up on the floor. Together, all those weights weighed as much as I did.

Not only that, but all of my reading and videos suggested that all the angles of one's limbs could vary greatly from person to person. Someone with a short torso, short arms, and long legs would look very different doing a deadlift than someone with long arms, long torso, and short legs.

The potential problems with deadlifts seemed to be many: hips shooting up, back rounding, bar drifting away from your legs, "squatting" the weight up instead of, well, deadlifting it. The even bigger problem was that my program only prescribed one set of deadlifts every week, which gave me only five measly reps to practice it. The book counseled that I had to be extremely careful to not exhaust my lower back with too many deadlift reps, which is why there were so few.

But because I got no practice time, I wasn't improving my form. They seemed to only strain my lower back more and more as I tried to add weight. I could technically get the bar up, and I kept hoping my form would develop alongside my progress. But I could feel my back getting pulled from a straight line into a curve, and the bar continued to drift out and away from my legs as I tried to will it back close to my body, where it wouldn't feel so heavy and out of control. Before I knew it, I was standing, however chaotically I'd gotten there, and another shitty rep was behind me, another opportunity to get it right, lost. Every once in a while, I'd get a session where everything felt right, where the weight didn't hang from my lower back or make me sore after, but I couldn't quite place exactly what was happening inside my body. And after five short reps, again it was over, a mystery that would carry over to yet another week.

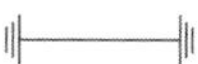

I needed another, lighter piece of equipment to take the place of the standard loaded barbell. I'd been making do with the fixed barbells arrayed in two A-frame stands—10, 20, 30, 40 pounds, all the way up to 120. To do my deadlifts, I would wrangle one of these smaller, fixed barbells off the A-frame and set it on the floor in front of a mirror. Because they were so small, the bar was much lower to the ground than the standard setup. I had to crunch myself down even more just to reach it, as if I were inviting another gym member to use me in a game of leapfrog.

Each time I went to deadlift one of these fixed barbells, I tried to casually look around me, first for anyone who appeared like they might be doing the same thing for me to imitate—no dice—and then for too-interested parties who, like Dimitrios, might be inclined to horn in on my amateur hour.

But everyone seemed focused on their own tasks. The ones who weren't lifting were drinking sports drinks, wiping sweat away, wiping down equipment, chatting with their friends.

One day, satisfied that I could test my best guess in peace, I tried to mimic the right movement, picking up the barbell in my hands and standing tall before trying to bend down until it hung approximately at mid-shin height before reversing back up.

Almost immediately, as if my pretend game of deadlifts had set off a silent alarm in the gym, a man materialized at my side, six feet tall with huge muscles to which clung his sweat-soaked T-shirt. "You should keep your legs straighter when you do that," he said. "Here—let me show you." Flustered, I stepped away from the barbell. He grabbed it and lowered it without bending his knees, then used the back of his legs and his lower back to pull himself up again. I didn't know much, but I knew this wasn't the deadlift I was looking for; it was a stiff-leg deadlift, a variation popular with bros who felt uncomfortable sticking their hips and butt out and back like a regular deadlift demanded. He didn't even care what I was actually trying to do.

"Like that," he said. "Now you try."

I withered inside at this forced performance for his benefit but did a couple noncommittal imitations of his movement, too fast, in a way that I hoped seemed indignant. "Okay, thanks. I get it now," I said.

"You know, I offer personal-training sessions," he said. So that's what he was after. I'd just wanted to do my workout, not fend off a sales pitch.

"Thanks, I'll keep that in mind," I said, putting my earbuds back in, praying that he wouldn't press me. He wandered away to another part of the gym, and I waited till he'd gotten a distance away before I breathed a sigh of relief. Even if he was gone, I felt once again like the gym was full of people to whom it was obvious that I did not belong. Most of them weren't coming up to yell it in my ear, but one was enough to remind me that I still wasn't exactly blending in.

In hopes it might make me look like I knew what I was doing, I replaced the 60-pound barbell and took a 70-pound one back to my spot and continued to seesaw the halves of my body up and down like a marionette. The deadlifts did not feel any better; if anything, the 70-pound weight seemed to be tugging on my lower back even more than the 60. But I was determined not to give even an inch to the interloping personal trainer, wherever he was perched like a gargoyle, presumably watching me struggle. I was annoyed at myself for trying to gracefully accommodate him and wanted to fight that impulse. But my desire to avoid conflict and keep quiet was proving more deep-seated than I realized.

It was somehow important to me that this guy not feel even a whit embarrassed for horning in on my session just to give me wrong information, and for forcing me to show I understood him, like a good little girl. It wasn't like I had to nuke him where he stood in retaliation for perceiving me, but I imagined it might feel good, even sanity-affirming, to not feel dragged by the heels into these kinds of interactions for once. I had way too much experience sublimating my end of them, bracing for metaphorical or literal strikes. I was always moving as if I might meet the business end of someone's explosive temper, or verbal, emotional, or physical abuse if I refused them attention.

I was sick of the self-abandonment. But to stop doing it, I'd have to do the opposite—once, for the first time—and somehow avoid being overwhelmed with guilt or regret or doubt. Like sticking my hand in a bag of eels as a trade for not having the bag dumped all over me. And then I'd have to do it again eventually, inevitably.

Any time I had to draw a line, I didn't feel like I was wrong at first. I had not planned on icing out my dad forever. I didn't really believe I was singularly responsible for his survival. But losing him was enough to make me distrust my own judgment. The raw smack of reality loomed over me, one big event among a million more that drove me inward to the only elements I felt I could truly control—my body, my food, the small daily life-giving or life-taking choices, meted out in the form of good or bad, reward or punishment. It was a weight I'd borne as if I deserved it. Now, I wanted release. But first I'd have to believe, myself, that I deserved release, and believe myself more than anyone else.

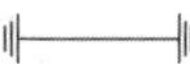

One of the last arguments with my recent ex-boyfriend had taken place one evening when we met in Midtown to see a play. I wore a dress I loved, red with navy stripes. In the bathroom, I assembled myself in selfie position in the mirror. I breathed in, puffing out my chest to suck my waist in and configure all my body parts for maximum thinness. I took the photo, put the phone back in my purse, and met him outside the bathroom. "You took a long time," he said. "What were you doing?"

"Taking a selfie," I said.

"Why?"

I paused. "I don't know," I said. "Because I wanted to."

"Let me see it." Reluctantly, I took my phone out of my purse, opened the photos, and showed him. He swiped through the multiple takes, Casey after Casey in the mirror, gaze directed downward, arms at angles. "Who was this for?" he said.

"What?" I said. "No one. I took it just to take it."

"Who did you send it to?"

"No one. There wasn't even time—"

"So you're going to send it later?" he said, handing the phone back to me with disdain, confident he'd uncovered the plot.

"*No*," I stressed as we walked into the theater. We sat down and the lights dimmed, but by the light of the stage I could see his agitation out of the corner of my eye. He fidgeted, folded creases in his program. My mind began to race, trying to think of an argument that might calm him down. He uncrossed and recrossed his legs, sighed. I began bracing, praying he'd calm down but running through the possible lines of defense and reasoning in my head. After twenty minutes, he abruptly stood up and walked out of the theater. I stayed in my seat: *Maybe he just went to the bathroom?* He didn't come back for the rest of the act.

When the lights went back up, I left the auditorium, looking around for him. He was leaning against the wall in a dark hallway that led to the foyer. He stood up as I approached. I thought maybe he'd say he was sorry, that he'd just needed a minute to collect himself. Instead, he started right in on me. "Why didn't you come see if I was okay? I was just *standing* out here—"

This was the worst: when the offenses started piling up on top of each other. Untangling them became impossible. Overwhelmed, I kept right on walking past him and ran down the two flights of stairs out to the street. I could hear him behind me, demanding me to stop, only managing to half form new interrogations before I got too far away for him to finish the sentence. I got across the street from the theater before he broke into a full sprint and caught up to position himself in front of me, still demanding me to stop, and I kept brushing past.

"Stop. Stop," he said. "Hold on. I'm trying to talk to you and you're not listening—"

He roughly grabbed my right arm. He had never grabbed me before. I looked up at his face and the moment dilated and spaghettified before me.

In engineering school, there are certain calculations you do over and over, to the point that the possible outcomes, the shortcuts, the numerical value of the constants become second nature. (If I had to look up the speed of light every time I had to use it in an equation, I'd have been in Physics III for a decade.)

In this moment, every rule I knew about men grabbing women flashed through my mind. The odds of it happening again, once it did. The possibility of de-escalation versus escalation. I'd been reading that book about abuse, hoping to learn how I could get him to stop; the book told me that I couldn't, that physical abuse often started late in the relationship and only escalated. I knew that retaliation or resistance was usually received poorly, at best. If I tried to remove my arm from his grip, I didn't know what might be coming. It scared me, the way that every time I tried to wrestle myself free, the knots just seemed to get tighter.

One option was to go limp. I could give in now, in the moment, to be safe. He lifted weights; he was much stronger than me, cardio-worn dinner-skipper, exhausted. Or I could risk it and resist and try to get away.

I tugged my arm away. He let it go but kept calling after me as I walked as fast as I could to the train. As I got farther and farther away, my mind became overwhelmed with the potential consequences of what I'd done, underscored by frustration at myself—how difficult this simple act of leaving an unwinnable argument had been. It was a kind of confusion and frustration I'd felt for years, the painful uncertainty over the cost of trying to give myself space and doing it wrong.

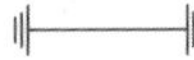

A few weeks after our argument outside the theater, my ex-boyfriend and I had broken up. I felt deep relief that that exchange hadn't gone a different way. But even as I finally reached the breaking point, I was miserable and uncertain. My body and brain were setting off every possible alarm over leaving, trying to protect me from making a choice I might possibly regret, that he might try to *make* me regret. I was so used to accepting responsibility, dancing more and more complex steps according to louder and louder and faster and faster music. But staying was hurting me, and much as my reflexes were driving me to take responsibility for him, those reflexes didn't serve me anymore. Holding it together was just a staunch refusal to admit that I was being hurt. The bathroom selfie remained in my phone, and when I scrolled back to it, I always found not myself but a slight-looking stranger who somehow didn't know the first thing about being fragile.

14

The Deadlift Cowgirls of Cyberspace

AS MISPLACED OR OBVIOUS as I sometimes felt in the gym, I was gradually becoming aware of a different kind of community that was completely changing how I thought about myself in relation to lifting weights. Not long before I started lifting in 2014, the set of tools available to new lifters had been very different. Only seven years before, my college campus didn't even have Wi-Fi throughout its buildings, and there were no iPhone cameras to film oneself at the gym, let alone social media apps to post to. The only way to understand what you looked like while lifting was to ask a fellow gym bro to watch you squat and then tell you what he thought. You had to hope, furthermore, that this random bro had any idea of what "good form" was—that is, the right way of doing the lift.

Form matters because it's meant to help bodies bend and move weights in the ways they are strongest and most likely to prevent injury. It's possible to pick up a heavy thing in all kinds of ways; the point of good form is to do it the way that won't leave us with a back injury. In the olden days, the rules of "good form" were contained in long, dense textbooks, where strength experts dedicated thousands of pages to documenting exactly what a good squat, or bench, or deadlift should look and feel like.

But over time, this textbook information filtered into gyms through a long game of Telephone from one bro to the next. A direction to "track one's knees over one's toes" in the Telephone pipeline might become "don't let your knees go past your toes." A direction to "sit back in one's hips" might become "keep the shins vertical." Strength-training scholarship suffered, and gyms entered an informational dark age. Before any of the bros knew it, most men had a godforsaken squat almost purpose-built to blow out their knees or throw out their lower back, even though they were trying their best. And it was a lot of men: even when I was in the right place—Richie's—I hardly ever saw any other beginner lifters, or even another woman, lifting.

And then smartphones happened. Good form was no longer only the provenance of people who cared to obtain, read, and interpret the technical language of dense strength-training texts like *Supertraining* or the Westside *Book of Methods*. A video was worth a million words. Once everyone had a camera in their pocket, it was easy for squatting experts to record themselves instructing squat mechanics for the whole world to see. Likewise, it was possible for anyone to record themselves squatting and send the video in the other direction, sharing it with a lot of people at once for feedback.

I didn't even dare attempt recording myself for several months, instead trying to see what I could in the mirrors (very little—it's impossible to have good form and watch the mirrors at the same time) and go by the new feelings trickling into my muscles. But feel wasn't enough for some of the problems: Was I "hitting depth," squatting deeply enough? Was my stance too wide, or not wide enough? Was my back straight? I had no real way of knowing, and while I felt more and more confident no one at Richie's was out for my blood, I didn't want to have to turn down any more personal-training sessions, either.

Eventually, curiosity about what my lifts looked like got the better of me. I captured a video on my phone, and there I was, squatting much better than I'd feared. I'd seen other people get "form checks" of their videos online, and so I posted a couple of mine to get feedback. "Looks good!" said most of the responses. "You're not always quite hitting depth, but you can get there. To fix your depth and butt wink, you could try doing some mobility stretches beforehand; it looks like your hamstrings are probably tight."

I started doing frog stretches before every session, resting face down on my spread knees and rocking my hips back, or pigeon poses, crooking one leg out in front while the other extended back behind me. Finding those stretches led me down more winding paths in the internet forest where I discovered that, while no one had really been looking, an online garden of powerlifting influencers had been growing on YouTube, on social media. And they seemed to represent everything I thought working out couldn't be.

These women loved lifting first and foremost—lived for it, even. They braided their exceptionally long protein-infused hair, put on booty shorts and a swingy crop top, laced up their Converse or Nike Romaleos, grabbed the barbell, and went to work. When they were in the gym, they were actually happy, checking off the boxes of their sets and reps, indulging in a little flex in the wall mirrors. After doing a particularly tough set of deadlifts—with her friend filming her, documentary style—a powerlifter might undo her lifting belt, throw it to a corner, crumple to the surface of the platform, and crawl away in a dramatic performance of exhaustion while the camera followed her, until she ultimately splayed flat on her back on the floor, one arm thrown across the top of her face, panting but smiling.

I was able to see all this in 2014 because lifters set their smartphones up on little tripods to film their reps from a quiet corner of the gym and then posted these videos to Instagram, which had only just started to allow video posts the year prior, in 2013. The women powerlifters posted their max attempts but also their fails, their accessory lifts, and their post-workout meals.

The really dedicated ones took to YouTube, where they could expound at length on not just their workouts and training goals, but the time between every training, when they busied themselves getting ready for the next training: eating, resting, trying out the latest massage foam roller or pressure-point cane. They detailed mixing their pre-workout shake, trying new protein powders, their meal preps, "full days of eating." They multi-tasked, drinking protein shakes while chopping vegetables, cooking rice, turning over marinated chicken or fish in a sauté pan, and combining it all into one big bowl they'd cover with ranch dressing or sriracha. The big food bowls would be followed by a helping of ice cream—sometimes the protein-infused diet brand meant to be eaten by the pint to get those last macros in, but often as not, some Ben & Jerry's.

One of my favorite lifters was named Meg and went by megsquats online. By day, she was a graphic designer; by night, she slung hundreds of pounds of iron. One of her earliest videos showed her pursuing a 300-pound squat by doing nothing but squatting for three months. As she continued to pursue lifting, she'd do things like holding open for the camera her Tupperware of meat-and-vegetable Bolognese she'd brought with her to work. She later opened up about the compulsive binge eating that followed her participation in a bikini body-building competition, describing the dieting and workouts as "really interesting, because it was so, so horrible…I really hated it, I hated it so bad."

After she left body building, she took up powerlifting, and in long videos, she would explain her powerlifting training: how she ate, how she was preparing for powerlifting meets she signed up for, what she put in her gym bag, which lifting shoes she wore. She explained that "if it fits your macros," you can eat it—a radically accepting approach that backlashed against the idea of there being good/bad, clean/unclean foods. She also used multiple videos to patiently explain a lifting program called the GZCL method to her followers. It was an arcane, higher-level approach that allowed the user to make a lot of customizations and, if they could be taught to wield it, gave them a lot of power. I inhaled these videos through the YouTube window.

What none of these women were concerned about was getting too big, an idea they laughed off with "Yeah, I wish." But instead of being dismissive, they understood the place from which the concern came and told their followers that nothing would happen to their bodies that wouldn't be within their control. It was as if what people thought, what other women thought, what men thought, simply didn't matter. In fact, most of them seemed to have found like-minded communities at their gym, people who were equally dedicated to and excited about training for strength. Women with the kinds of bodies I'd never seen on magazine covers—muscular but not body-building-stage lean, fit but not Pilates-willowy. These unconventional-looking women ruled Instagram with tens or hundreds of thousands of followers, existing in a kind of harmonious bliss, relishing all these aspects of living that I'd always only grimly endured.

Many of them were exceptionally strong, on their way to elite competitions like the International Powerlifting Federation's world competition, or the USAPL nationals, or "the Arnold," an invite-only competition at a yearly festival held by Schwarzenegger himself.

But just as many had no particular ambition. And that, to me, was the most fascinating part of all. I was used to the visible athletes being the ones who possessed otherworldly talent—the fastest, the strongest, the most cunning on the field or with a ball in their hands. I was used to self-affirmation being wrapped up in accomplishment and achievement. But these women weren't getting attention because they were the best of the best, or because they were aiming to be. And even though they were doing all of these things that they "shouldn't," they weren't doing backflips to justify themselves or make excuses for their choice of sport, how they looked, what they ate. I was so used to seeing women defend or apologize for these kinds of choices, especially if they weren't for the purpose of being hotter and getting toned, or "losing weight" to be "healthier." They had found something better, something they loved, and it had made them throw off the chains and forget about everything that came before.

They weren't "real" people in any material sense to me; I didn't really know them and didn't really know anyone like them. But the portal that opened up inside of my phone made me feel less alone when I actually *was* alone as the only woman using the weights in my gym; they made me feel not crazy for wanting to eat, for wanting to grow, for not finding ultimate satisfaction in dieting and yoga/Pilates/cardio. While the facts of lifting and eating had toppled everything I knew about my body, this handful of social media accounts had toppled everything I thought was true about the perception and culture of people who did this lifting and eating. They existed, even as my real-life environment failed to produce them, and even as the media that purported to represent the interests of my incredibly mainstream demographic failed to represent them.

15

The Untold Story of American Strength

AS I SAW MORE people—a variety of people—lifting weights for different reasons, I wanted to pinpoint exactly why I had been so on edge about joining Richie's in the first place. What had shaped my prejudices? I saw some of my thinking reflected in a 2014 piece for the magazine *Pacific Standard* titled "How the Other Half Lifts: What Your Workout Says About Your Social Class," where writer Daniel Duane described his experience with starting to lift heavy weights. He explained how much his perception of his body had changed for the better when he got stronger: "My strength numbers shot upward, and so did my body weight: 190 pounds, 200, 210, 215," he wrote. "Walking down the sidewalk, I felt confident. At parties with my wife, I saw men who ran marathons, and they looked gaunt and weak. I could have squashed them."

Unfortunately, his family and peers looked down on his lifting: at best they were confounded and at worst put off by his new interest, which scanned to them as threatening, even low-class. "The so-called dominant classes… especially those like my friends and myself, richer in fancy degrees than in actual dollars—tend to express dominance through strenuous aerobic sports that display moral character, self-control, and self-development, rather than physical dominance," he wrote. "By chasing pure strength, in other words, packing on all that muscle, I had violated the unspoken prejudices—and dearly held self-definitions—of my social group." Duane's wife even admitted that, for reasons she didn't or couldn't articulate, she was more attracted to him when he was smaller, compared to his bulkier weight-training physique. Eventually, Duane gave up the weights to become a triathlete, but he lamented his choice. "No matter what I'm supposed to feel about physical dominance or moral character," he wrote, "I dearly miss feeling huge walking down the street."

In my own experience, there was a cultural perception of bigger, stronger women as unattractive, even abhorrent, that I felt a lot of pressure to believe. Going back to the Saturday-morning cartoons of my youth, it felt like Bugs Bunny and Pepé Le Pew and Yosemite Sam were always going gaga over the irresistibly demure, unassuming female characters, and ran from the big, strong, loud ones so fast that they left flaming tire tracks. The latter characters were almost always not just unattractive but also overconfident, un-self-aware, too loud.

Upon diving in to research this phenomenon, I felt certain I could have imagined or at least inflated it in my memory. Then I stumbled upon a TV Tropes page for the "Brawn Hilda" character archetype that precisely described what took root so firmly in my child brain: "a strong, mannish, usually foreign woman…her strength is seen as unattractive, as she usually (purposely or not) 'emasculates' the hero by beating him up or outdoing him in 'manly' activities…The vast majority of the time her personality is irrelevant: She's just a gag character whose humor stems from being the opposite of a hot exotic chick." It's not limited to cartoons, either: the page lists hundreds of examples and isn't even exhaustive—it lacks one of the most indelible Brawn Hildas of my own time, Big Rhonda from *That '70s Show*, but does include another, Big Patty of *Hey Arnold!*

What did it mean when Duane's wife preferred him to be small? What did it mean for Duane himself to miss feeling huge, even as he capitulated to a "trendier" appearance? Why did I believe that being "bulky" was bad, even threatening, to my livelihood and success as a woman? Why were "long, lean" body types and endurance sports cherished by non-working-class people, while stronger-looking bodies were reviled? How did physical might, either in appearance or function, become tangled up in so many widely disdained characteristics?

I had a sense that lifting weights belonged only to already-strong people, but especially people for whom strength seemed tightly interlaced with their work: military and paramilitary organizations, or jobs that required physical labor. Yet that logic didn't apply across other forms of working out; I didn't consider cardio fitness to belong only to, say, bike messengers, or chiseled cores to belong only to ballerinas. I wanted to understand why strength was so stigmatized.

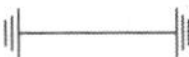

Of course, physical training in some form or another goes back to ancient times. The origin of our modern conception of working out with weights is often pegged to something called the Muscular Christianity movement of America in the mid-1800s. I could see how lifting as an outgrowth of a religious initiative would be off-putting to, say, Daniel Duane's intellectual family. But I was surprised to learn that there was also a little-known history to our modern concept of physical activity as a voluntary but essential and empowering part of maintaining health (as opposed to an obligatory part of, say, running a subsistence farm).

This approach to exercise began with a bunch of socialist-minded Germans who loved to lift heavy things. They were called the Turners. This is the story of how a gym teacher and strength training led to a national network of gyms for the people in the United States.

The Turners were named after the founder of the Turner movement, the "Turnvater," Friedrich Ludwig Jahn. In 1809, Jahn was a humble but idealistic gym teacher in the city of Berlin. Jahn hated that the French, especially Napoleon, were constantly trying to take over the German confederation of states. He attributed the states' vulnerability, in part, to the impoverished minds and bodies of the German populace. As gym teachers are wont to do, he thought maybe, just maybe, the people could reinvigorate their minds, and thereby their spirits, and thereby their pride and independence, through physical activity.

By 1811, Jahn had built an open-air gymnasium in Berlin named Turnplatz—basically a giant playground for grown-ups. It was ostensibly a place to practice gymnastics, vaulting, tumbling, acrobatics, and other feats of strength. But Jahn also made sure everyone who might visit had their eyes on the prize: preserving German culture and protecting it from the outside influence of the dreaded French. Jahn gave talks on German culture, led groups in the singing of German songs, and scheduled contests with awards around culturally German holidays. In 1828, Jahn published *A Treatise on Gymnasticks*, a 235-page instruction manual on every exercise movement he cared to document, including "pushing," "lifting" instruments to measure strength, "carrying," and "exercises with dumb-bells."

In 1848, the Turner gymnasts banded together and fought for the German revolution, but without many weapons or men, they were crushed by Prussian troops. Eventually, the Turners in Germany were prevented from gathering, and their gyms were dismantled.

Many of the Turners then made their way to America over the next couple of decades. In this new and developing country, they became strong advocates for public physical education, but also for "controversial" causes, including abolition and socialism. The Turner Union's main enemy was oppression, and they resolved to fight any power that infringed on individual rights on the basis of skin color, gender, or place of birth. They opposed religious influence in government, including tax exemption for churches or using religious phrases on government currency or documents. The Turners supported the Republican political party of Abraham Lincoln in the lead-up to and during the Civil War, and many joined up as Union soldiers. Turners repeatedly served as Lincoln's bodyguards, including during his inauguration.

When they arrived in America, the Turners set about building "Turner halls," or Turnverein, some of which still stand in the US today, where they held regular "Turnfests" (athletic events). While they loved athletic displays, the Turners grew to abhor the American fixation on competitions and records: they felt winning spoiled young people, encouraged individualism, and discouraged actual, equitable physical education.

Turner clubs grew into a meeting place for working-class immigrants, and a particular interest of the Turners was fighting for better labor conditions. One man named August Spies was a leader of the 1886 Haymarket labor demonstration in support of an eight-hour workday. That demonstration turned into a massacre and, in the aftermath, was used against the labor movement, but it ultimately fueled activism against grueling work schedules and led to the institution of the eight-hour workday. Spies was the editor of a radical labor-driven newspaper, a union supporter, and a Turner.

The Turner movement peaked in 1893 with a membership of over forty thousand people. There were nine Turner halls in St. Louis alone (more than the current number of Planet Fitnesses, YMCAs, and CrossFits combined in the city today). The movement was rooted in immigrant communities in a country with a strong bent toward assimilation, so its influence eventually faded. But the Turners reveal an undeniably communal and collective foundation for our American conception of exercise culture, especially when it came to recreational strength.

The Turners saw health as a right for every person. They saw it not just as a matter of ability, but a vector for collective care, for spreading equitable power among the people, not just to enrich their individual lives but to help them stand together against those who would potentially enslave or exploit them. They valued the power of the individual, not as an island, but as a link in the chain. To the extent that each could give according to his ability, the Turners saw it as their duty to protect the less powerful and raise the floor for every person.

I was charmed by the wholesome idea of sweet, earnest socialists sharing their benches and plates, locking their buff arms in solidarity against forces that benefitted from separating them, isolating them, or manipulating them into competing with one another over scraps. How sad that this activity had now become enveloped in machismo, the pursuit of being "alpha," aesthetics, and establishing dominance. I resolved to dig more; I wanted to know exactly what had brought this utopian association down for good.

16

A Perfect Online Storm

I PASSED THE SUMMER of 2014 visiting Richie's three times a week, happily alternating my sets with rests and downing a bounty of hot-weather foods. Burgers, hot dogs, fried dough and clam strips at Coney Island. Boldly flavored ice creams of new trendy parlors: miso cherry, Earl Grey tea, maple bacon pecan, cardamom lemon jam. I tried to get my workouts in early in the day before the humid weather started to challenge Richie's air-conditioning, sometimes creating an indoor tropical microclimate that slicked the floor with condensation. This allowed me to shower and settle in, to shelter against the heat for the rest of the day as I blogged.

Over Labor Day weekend, some hackers dumped a truly staggering number of nude and lascivious photos of celebrities directly onto the internet. The Fappening, as it came to be called (from the verb "to fap," online slang for "masturbating"), happened while I was at a Labor Day weekend party.

"Wait," said my friend Linda, tapping around on her phone. "There's a bunch of celebrity nude photos? Just *on* the internet?" The silent question in everyone's mind became whether it would be too weird to also pick up their phones, in front of everyone else, and seek out the photos themselves. The game theory of it staggered most of us into inaction, relying on the reports of a few people who had first happened upon the story.

Curiosity got the better of me by the time I got home. Many websites were already making efforts to prevent users from posting the photos on forums or as threads on Reddit, less out of a sense of propriety than out of fear of getting sued. But as a tech culture reporter, this might cross into my coverage area; I couldn't report blind. After some maneuvers, I was able to find a few of the photos: fully nude Jennifer Lawrence, Krysten Ritter posing cheekily with a couple of different salads.

I closed the tabs, my skin crawling. There had already been lively online debate around the role of celebrities in our lives, their increasing ubiquity (as a result of social media) fostering what we came to call parasociality, a highly one-sided relationship that led us to feel a lot closer to them than the other way around. *Celebrities are not your friends*, went one side of the argument; *we don't have to defend them from any and all criticism. They're not going to love you back*. And then the rejoinder from the other side: *Celebrities are people, too.*

The hack had also come directly on the heels of a culture clash that had been the subject of much scrutiny in the tech world, as well as my workplace. It came to be known as Gamergate, where a bunch of online bottom dwellers, fed up with rising discourse over misogyny and prurience in video games as a medium, realized that they could band together. They aired their grievances under the guise of "ethics in games journalism" and began threatening the livelihoods of the people and publications they thought were the worst offenders.

Gamergaters filled the email inboxes of executives at companies who advertised on game-journalism websites, accusing the editors and writers of "unethical behavior" over, for instance, critiquing a game with too much misogynistic violence, or praising a game for featuring LGBTQ issues or characters. This would cause the companies to pull their ads from these sites, cutting off publications' financing. Gamergaters also began a terror campaign targeting people they saw as enemies, including game developer Zoë Quinn, doxing her personal information and hacking her various online accounts, after one of her exes wrote a delusional blog post claiming game critics were soft on her due to her gender. Anita Sarkeesian, a video game critic who often analyzed games through the lens of gender studies, was avalanched with threats of rape and death until she notified the police.

Gamergaters justified their harassment as nothing more than a passionate defense of the video games they loved. But the intensity and tactics were not equal to the stated cause of "video game journalists shouldn't weigh in on gender politics." The under- and overtones were clear: marginalized groups and women who didn't know their place in the video game world had better watch it, or else. If someone found the representation of women in video games degrading or offensive, be it their tiny, ineffectual pieces of armor or fawning, insubstantial dialogue, that wasn't just their opinion. It was an assault on the sanctity of gaming tradition.

If this seems familiar, it's because these kinds of tactics and rhetoric set a template for many future wars waged by a paranoid conservative fringe to protect a discriminatory status quo: on "wokeism," on "diversity, equity, and inclusion." It was Gamergate that gave rise to the use of "social justice" and "social justice warrior" (SJW) as pejorative terms.

Days before the Fappening, high on the empowerment I'd been feeling from lifting weights and returning to my body, I'd written a spirited attack on the warped logic Gamergaters used to justify their attacks on women. The article performed extremely well, and colleagues from other websites complimented my straight shooting in the face of some of the internet's most vitriolic and deranged users. The piece garnered over eighteen hundred comments, a staggering number even for our kibitzy site—suggesting at least a few people thought I was wrong, and even more wanted to argue about the nuances of why and how I was wrong, or not. The going advice to online writers was to never, under any circumstances, read the comments. I virtually always did (hoping for the positive responses to wash over me like a soothing wave, only to be dragged under by worrying over the negative comments, no matter how few there were). This time, though, I never even opened the comments section.

Still, when it came to the subject of gender politics, my editors had suddenly cautioned me on the importance of remaining "objective," a concern that had never really been central to our coverage. They knew their audience, especially some of its most vocal members, were less than progressive on this issue. That was to say nothing of their own politics (one of the editors had once declared he'd physically assault anyone who initiated a conversation on gender pronouns, a sentiment met with zero pushback from the rest of the leadership). I assured them not to worry; I felt straight on the facts. And I did. A lot of publications chose to equivocate about Gamergate: one side says this, the other side says that; we can exclusively confirm that the two sides disagree.

But I knew the intensity of the vitriol, and the choice of target, was a backlash over more than whether female characters' armor was practical enough. I didn't want to hedge in order to soothe the people who resisted these basic truths. And I didn't want to capitulate to degenerates who spent their time making women's lives hell because the women thought selling a game called *Moon War* using a woman dressed in a Hooters uniform was a bit much.

The editors preferred the style of an article written by one of my coworkers, a security reporter covering the technical details of the Fappening. Though no one yet knew exactly how the photos had been obtained, he wrote a lengthy piece on the basics of cloud storage, where exactly files go, and how they are protected. "Caveat Self-or," he proclaimed in the last section, an awkward play on "caveat emptor," or "buyer beware." "Anyone should take pause before disrobing before their smartphone camera—regardless of the phone operating system or how that image will be delivered to its intended audience."

His article caused a mild backlash, both among readers and some of our staff. The writer offered to take any feedback anyone had. I wrote to him, saying it sounded like victim blaming. "From a purely security-focused standpoint," he responded, "'caveat selfor' is, I believe, a sound piece of advice—not victim blaming." I tried again, explaining that telling people not to use a ubiquitous service from an established company was not very helpful at all. "You asked people to give you cogent feedback on why this is victim blaming, and I'm telling you," I said. He, and our editors, dismissed me.

It seemed blindingly obvious why it was wrong to lay the blame on the subjects of the photos, as opposed to the hackers. Sure, I knew a different set of rules governed the privacy of public figures, but the discourse around the Fappening appeared particularly sinister and somehow connected to the bloodthirstiness of Gamergate. Yet I still felt horribly unequal to these moments, trying to advocate for what I thought was right but plagued with doubt about how certain everyone else seemed. They seemed as comfortable ignoring me as I was uncomfortable raising an objection. When they didn't hear me, I regretted even trying.

17

Hold Your Breath

THE FIRST POWERLIFTING MEET I ever saw I happened upon by accident in the streets of Brooklyn. One Saturday a few months into my own lifting practice, I took the long way home from a friend's apartment. On the way, I found myself on a block where people were spilling out of a completely open storefront. Music playing from inside pounded through the air. As I drew closer, I realized people were thronged around a couple of platforms set up inside. Upon the various platforms were setups for a bench rack, a barbell, and plates.

There were several rows of chairs inside, and because some were on risers, the room felt packed not just side to side, but floor to ceiling. By now, I'd seen videos online of people competing with the camera trained on the lifters, and while it was possible to hear distant-sounding cheers off-screen, the events always seemed relatively chaste, on the level of a golf tournament: a slow procession of lifters. Here in person, though, at a small gym on a side street in a little-populated part of the city, the noise could have been mistaken for a wrestling or football match.

The crowd seemed as if it was genuinely trying to bring down the building. They were gaga for these lifters, in thrall to every step of the process repeated for each person. Even among the chairs, most people were on their feet, shouting—yells of encouragement as the lifter got set up, screams of "UP! UP!" I stopped and watched as one woman after another approached the bench in turn, unracked the bar with the help of volunteers, and pumped out bench reps as the crowd went crazy.

Judges lined the perimeter of the stage, and when one judge in front would call out, "Start," the lifter would lower the bar to their rib cage, holding it there until the judge called out, "Press," when they would force it back up into the air—150, 175, 200 pounds.

"Rack," the judge would say when they'd fully extended their arms, and the volunteers would help them snap the barbell back to its hooks. The woman would then pop up from the bench, and the crowd would go wild as everyone watched a set of three lights to the side of the stage that would flicker on in various combinations, indicating whether each judge had passed or failed them. Two or three white lights was a good lift (causing the crowd to stomp and scream a second time). With one or zero white lights, the lift was disqualified ("aws" and sighs of disappointment, followed by encouraging clapping).

Because the gym was so small, I was both barely inside and also only a few feet from the platform myself, along with several other onlookers. But we didn't even register to the lifters, who were absolutely laser focused on the task at hand. As I stood there, one lifter approached the setup in a singlet patterned like the night sky, spangled with stars and colorful clouds of galactic matter. She sat down on the bench, deftly adjusting the wraps on her wrist, before twisting around at the midback to reach one hand back to the barbell, then arching into a backbend to reach the other hand back and slowly lower her shoulders down to the padded bench, such that there was enough space to fit a football under her back between her butt and shoulder blades. The volunteers lifted the barbell into her hands, and the crowd bellowed as she pursed her lips with effort and lowered the 165 pounds to her chest. "Press," said the judge, and her face reddened as the bar glided smoothly back into the air. Once it was racked, she popped up and un-Velcro'd her wraps, her eyes on the lights, her feet dancing lightly. All three lights turned white—the lift was good. The crowd exploded with cheers, the woman pumped her fist, then strode through the curtains that obscured the back of the gym. In a moment, another woman in a singlet emerged from the curtains, marching out with equal determination.

The whole event was a lot to take in. The meet was presided over by an exceptionally tall man holding a microphone who was dressed, for all intents and purposes, as if he'd been imported straight from a pirate-themed amusement park: bandanna wrapped over his long hair; long-tailed black coat; slim pants with a red sash; earrings; fingerless gloves; and not a little black eyeliner. This was Geno, a fixture of the powerlifting scene who made a point of emceeing as many events as he could around the world. But for his size and spectacle, he emceed the meet with grace, crossing nimbly back and forth in what little space was left.

"Here comes Ms. Toya Gomez with her third bench attempt. She stands to pull into first place if she can pull off her 235 pounds, but after failing her first two attempts at 195 and 215, she has a challenge ahead of her. Lifter ready…and…it's good! Ms. Gomez pulls into first place, but she's not in the clear yet. Here comes Claire Constantine through the warm-up curtain—"

I stayed for a while, watching lifters cycle in and out. For each, the volunteers added or subtracted plates before reassembling around the rack to carefully spot, moving with the weight to catch it in case she faltered. And some women did—the barbell would come to rest on their chests and fail to move again or make it only a few inches up before collapsing back down. Sometimes the barbell took an unsteady path, swerving or even retreating back down before ultimately rising into the air. Unfortunately, this disqualified the lift: only lifts that kept upward momentum counted. But the spotters would sweep the weight away as if it weren't weight at all, and the lifter would spring back up, on to thinking about her next attempt. Every lifter reflected the basic pattern of a good lift: square up, take the weight, breathe, brace, hold tension, release tension, rerack the weight.

Ever since before I could remember, I've habitually held my breath and been unable to breathe normally (at least while I'm conscious). This habit is unnoticeable to me, like some kind of waking sleep apnea, until I remember to check and almost always realize I'm doing it. Counter to the expression "so quiet she didn't even breathe," it was always somehow incredibly loud to my mother. I'd be sitting and watching TV and my mom would tap me on the arm. "Stop holding your breath," she'd chide me.

In running, the ideal breathing pace is a measured inhale through the nose, followed by a slighter, slower exhale through the mouth. Two steps to take a breath in, three steps to breathe out, repeat. But during running, too, I struggled to breathe regularly. It didn't help that the more pain I was in, the more I seemed to hold my breath—which would cause more pain in the form of cramps.

But in lifting weights, the breathing is much more structured, not just to get oxygen but to make the whole physical movement work. It's organized the same way as the rest of the lift is—building tension with which to create force, followed by release.

Each lifting rep starts by first taking a breath—not a belly-deep one, just enough to fill the lungs most of the way. But that breath is not just a breath; the air becomes a key structural element in the physical act of doing the lift. By filling our insides with air, we give our core something to grip around, which helps solidify what would otherwise be an overly flexible midsection. Gripping on to this breath, or "bracing," as it's called in the sport of powerlifting, prevents most movements from turning into a heave of the tiny lower back muscles. The breath becomes a tool: it helps stabilize the spine and turns the passive, bendy core into an active asset.

To keep the breath in, we close the airway and press the breath against the inside of that closed airway. This part is known as the Valsalva maneuver (if you've ever strained to get a bowel movement out, you've probably Valsalva'd without knowing it). During a Valsalva maneuver, bodies aren't just holding breath; the act of Valsalva'ing actually helps manage blood flow to make muscles more effective.

It produces a brief rise in blood pressure, which the body responds to by reducing heartbeat frequency. As a result, blood pressure then drops for the next ten to fifteen seconds, for most people idling well below baseline, while the rate of their heartbeat slowly increases. When the breath is released, blood rushes back into the heart, blood pressure rises, and the heartbeat falls again.

The metaphor coaches tell lifters to imagine with bracing and Valsalva'ing is that of a soup can, like we are turning our torso into a solid cylinder. We hold on to that breath through the course of the rep, and at the end, exhale. Before the next rep, we take another breath and repeat the whole process. Most of the muscles we think of as "the core" are relatively small, but using them together in this specific way makes them greater than the sum of their parts. This was what every lifter in the meet was doing on every lift: breathing in, holding, breathing out.

After a while, all the lifters had made all of their bench attempts, and the meet paused as volunteers began maneuvering the bench setup off to one side. Now they were bringing in a deadlift jack, a long handle with two pronged forks on each end that could lift the barbell off the floor to slide plates on and off. The crowd quieted to a murmur of in-group conversations and checking of phones. I'd already ended up watching the din for a solid half hour, and now I was running late. I backed out of the crowd that now spilled even more onto the sidewalk, and returned to the sunny street.

As I left, I was bursting with hard-charging feeling; I'd never seen that before. Women as strong as that, performing solo on a stage, unapologetically flexing all their might. They seemed so completely focused and inside the task that faced them, as unusual a task as it was. Not only that, but everyone in the room was entirely behind them. I was so used to watching myself carefully and skeptically, expecting that others were watching me carefully and skeptically, if at all. But I had never really recognized the ambient skeptical, even disdainful, gaze that almost always clouded my reality, until I felt it completely gone from that room. Unlike even a regular women-focused sporting event (if there could be said to be such a thing), the spirit of the thing seemed not to critique or to measure. The idea was to get fucking wild and shoot the moon, to let women set the terms of their personal best and throw themselves unbridled at achieving or blowing past it or, maybe more importantly, failing to do so. Even as I'd played and followed women's sports myself, I'd never seen or felt this energy before.

Up until I had turned onto that corner and watched the meet, I had believed that competing in lifting was always going to be a bridge too far for me and that I was content to just go to the gym, do my training, notch my little weight increases, and go home. But now I was completely enthralled with that environment and the purity of the community's spirit I'd observed. It wasn't about winning; it wasn't about failing—it was simple, uninhibited enjoyment of their own and each other's physicality. Even heading away from the crowd and down the block, I was convinced—there was no way I couldn't eventually give competing a shot.

18

The Struggle for American Strength

I RETURNED TO RICHIE'S with even more zeal than I already had for lifting. The powerlifting meet I'd encountered had taken my strength-building experience that had been happening only in my head and body and dragged it literally out onto the street. I was not nearly as alone as I sometimes felt, nor was I alone in how it affected my relationship to the world. I was thrilled to unexpectedly see it reflected back at me even more intensely than I felt it. There was a real, live "we," and I wanted to throw myself into training even harder as a result in order to follow this thread I'd accidentally pulled. As alienated as I'd felt by lifting and gym culture as it appeared to me from the outside, I was delighted to discover from the inside that the actual practice of it couldn't be more different. It begged the question, again, of how the "through-the-looking-glass" version of lifting could be and feel so much better than the warped, intimidating version I'd previously seen and believed.

When I had dug around trying to understand our cultural relationship with lifting weights, I'd instantly connected it with what I'd learned about the Turners and their vast network of gymnasiums—a benevolent society of kind juggernauts promoting strength as a resource for a community, health as a public good. This resonated with what I'd found in my own new experience of my body and my gym. And yet, this dynamic didn't at all describe how the average person interpreted a weight room here and now: as a competition for dominance, machismo, intimidation, elitism. I couldn't help but feel that strength had somehow been co-opted and siloed. How had this happened? I dove back into researching to find out.

While the Turners were enjoying their American communities and pursuing physical feats of strength over the course of the 1800s, Christian leaders in the US were noticing that their congregations had developed a manliness problem. The Christian men of society, they felt, had grown too soft. Like good Christians, they knew how to suffer and deny their physical impulses; like good Victorian gentlemen, they knew how to talk about books and art and other "civilized" topics. But as future president Theodore Roosevelt fretted publicly in 1899: there was no one to protect the United States from a growing threat of oversentimentality. Not only that, but church service attendance had begun to skew up to 75 percent female. Wherever the men were, they were not in church reflecting on ways to best serve the Lord.

It wasn't only Christians who were worried, either. Scientists were troubled by a pall that had settled over the modern world. After the onset of the Industrial Revolution in the late 1700s, people became much more aware of their limits, thanks to new methods of measuring and optimizing their productivity. This was exacerbated when they compared unfavorably to the new, inexhaustible machines that had wormed their way into the production process in many industries. People seemed to be newly tired or ailing, and the presumed cause was too much mental or physical work. Health experts had begun to discourage strenuous exercise in the mid to late 1800s because it would cause the development of "parasitic muscles." Yet the cause of this new condition that gripped so many couldn't solely be overwork—it struck down even relatively well-off urban dwellers. These wealthy city folks' needs were more than met, and they didn't suffer for food or a secure place to sleep. They might work, but not too much; if anything, they worked sparingly. And yet, they also seemed to be slipping into a dark place, a place of pain, a place of hopelessness. They were weak and didn't want to leave bed, dizzy, even prone to fainting. The New York physician George Miller Beard dubbed the condition "neurasthenia" in the 1860s.

At that time, neurasthenia was a new, wide-ranging diagnosis meant to capture "all the forms of and types of exhaustion coming from the brain." In his sociological case study, *Suicide*, Emile Durkheim wrote that for neurasthenics, "every movement [is] an exertion…the performance of physiological functions is a source of generally painful sensations." Doctors were unsure how exactly to effectively treat neurasthenia, but they tried to triangulate a unifying causal theory: it seemed to be some problem with modernity, industrialization, disconnection.

German economist Karl Bücher proposed that labor was actually beneficial to human bodies, and that this malaise had something to do with the lack of opportunities for bodily "rhythm" that was normally provided by manual labor: hauling, threshing, carrying, heaving and ho'ing. But this theory depended on human beings being the ones to determine tempo of movement and when to stop—not the machines. Unfortunately, the demands of the machines that were increasingly used were not calibrated to the people running them; people could only adjust to, try to keep up with, the machines. Labor became something machines did, not befitting the "thinking" man. And since machines didn't have to be paid and could be unilaterally implemented (unless laborers managed to object or strike), the powerful few became the arbiters of this devaluation of human labor.

As for the ailing Christians, something had to change. A Christian reverend named Charles G. Finney had begun reaching for an answer in 1837, in a lecture called "Christian Perfection":

> Christian perfection is a duty,…[Christians] may think they are willing to be perfect, but they deceive themselves…there are many sins they are unwilling to give up…Have you not, beloved, known times when one great absorbing topic has so filled your mind, and controlled your soul, that the appetites of the body remained, for the time, perfectly neutralized? Now, suppose this state of mind to continue, to become constant; would not all these physical difficulties be overcome, which you speak of as standing in the way of perfect sanctification?

From this concept of Christian perfection and Charles G. Finney, Muscular Christianity of the 1900s blossomed. As educational philosopher G. Stanley Hall put it in an address to a Boston YMCA in 1901, "We would bring in a higher kingdom of man, regenerate in body…Men are, happily, just now beginning to learn what a power can be brought to bear against the kingdom of evil in the world by right body keeping."

Hall was, in fact, looking at the Turners specifically as inspiration. To exist as a fine specimen of man, Hall reasoned, was a credit to the goodness of God. This translated well to the realm of sports in general: God also loved teamwork, cooperation, loyalty, and respect for authority. If religion could be an opiate of the masses, it could also be a drill sergeant, whipping its constituents into a formidable standing army.

Muscular Christianity was a movement that emphasized masculinity, athleticism, and discipline. It had no formal founder or leadership, but it resonated with the Christian Protestantism that underpins our American love of hard work and dovetailed with a drive for self-improvement.

The possibility of manifesting heaven on earth through good works and personal perfection created a groundswell of interest. It was Muscular Christianity that gave us the Young Men's Christian Association's push for the physical well-being of "the whole man," when it started to include physical recreation programming for all YMCAs in 1864. To these groups, physical strength and capability were no longer a collective social good; they were mandates in service of God. By 1874, there were nearly four hundred YMCA gyms in the United States, and in 1881, a YMCA staffer coined the term "body building."

The unofficial periodical of the Muscular Christianity movement was *Physical Culture*, a magazine that started as pages and pages of text and later evolved into a glossy book of illustrations and photos. *Physical Culture* urged its readers, often in near paroxysms of prose, toward their perfectible physical, and therefore moral, religious, and philosophical, destiny. While *Physical Culture* was less directly religious than the sermons and writings that pushed serving God with physical strength, what it lacked in piety it made up for in macho broadsides.

"It is the editor's firm and conscientious belief," wrote editor Bernarr A. Macfadden in the first volume published in 1900, "that weakness is a crime. That one has no more excuse for being weak than he can have for going hungry when food is at hand…The finest and most satisfying results that can be acquired from proper physical culture are the cure of disease and the development of that energy, vitality and health essential to the success and happiness of life."

Physical Culture was popular with the Muscular Christians, but in fact, the publication had taken the Muscular Christianity philosophy that men had to be fit in order to be perfect and best serve God and lopped off the "serve God" part. By doing that, it landed on a rhetoric that leveraged the religious power of belief for the intoxicating possibility of total personal agency—via mastery over one's physicality.

For someone who felt insecure or cast aside for their supposed faults of weakness and imperfection to suddenly hear a voice booming down from on high (or from the pages of a magazine) that with enough effort, they could become strong, vigorous, perfect—that was catnip to anyone steeped in the American values of hard work, achievement, and individualism.

The trend of physical culture and Muscular Christianity faded out around the time of World War I almost two decades later, which forced the realization that military might had far less to do with physical power and much more to do with the size and number of its guns. But physical strength was dragged out again when it came time to symbolize the power and discipline of fascist regimes.

Physical culture found its way back to Germany again in the 1930s in the form of government-sponsored fitness campaigns, where it was again politicized but this time used to intimidate and stratify. The fascist association with physical training was so powerful that similar programs in Great Britain foundered; no one wanted to work out like fascists did in Germany and Italy.

From then on, exercise never again achieved the populist or socialist associations that brought it to the United States in the first place; once Christian, capitalist, and even fascist propagandists hooked their claws into it, they didn't let go. When it came to lifting weights, specifically, the culture split into two directions. One was aesthetic, the culture of body building, symbolized by the rise of figures like Jack LaLanne and Joe Weider and, eventually, Arnold Schwarzenegger.

The other was more functionally driven and militaristic. In 1942, during World War II, the army introduced a physical-fitness test: squat jumps, sit-ups, pull-ups, push-ups, and a three-hundred-yard run. The rest of the military and, eventually, local and state law enforcement departments began requiring physical-fitness tests as part of their application process.

Then in 1960, John F. Kennedy published an article in *Sports Illustrated* titled "The Soft American" that, like Jahn before him, lamented the weak physical resolve of his country. Unlike Jahn, Kennedy was motivated by Cold War panic. This set the stage for the Presidential Physical Fitness Test instituted in 1966 as a way of trying to enforce fitness among the nation's youth, the better to staff the US military.

Today, weight-training sports still keep close associations with the military and law enforcement. These ties have given rise to the perception of lifting as a tool of fascism or elitism, or as service to a higher power, instead of where its real origins lie, as envisioned by the Turners: a public social good that unites and empowers the collective of civilians *against* imperialism, capitalism, and fascism.

If the Turners are any evidence, it was beneficial for capitalists to keep equitable physical education away from the hands of the average person, lest it help them feel enabled to stand with each other against oppression, as the Turners did. With a few moves over only a hundred or so years, powerful entities—successful capitalists, Christianity, fascists, militarists—co-opted the collective modern tradition of physical training and capability into one that served them. They made subservience to power into the only logical, sensical reason to have individual personal strength. This cast laborers as dumb, lower-class, and less-than. Why would you bother being strong if you don't have to physically serve someone else?

This idea then worked its way upward, such that any outward signs of performing physical labor—muscles, sweat—became distasteful to display. It's why writer Daniel Duane's family felt uncomfortable with his new size and shape—their cultural programming alerted them that he was behaving outside of his class, in a way that challenged the status quo. They had internalized the messaging that strength's place is in service of power. Strength is a marker of being a (good) servant. Physical power to serve the powerful, for the enforcement of the powerful and reinforcement of the existing power structures: good, appropriate, sensical. Physical power developed for other reasons: bad, off-putting, distasteful, wrong, and worst of all, challenging to the status quo.

This goes double for women, whose bodies are already maniacally scrutinized and controlled. Enforcing the importance of diet and weight loss literally keeps everyone, especially women, in a weakened state. Therefore, actually gaining strength is a stacked threat. Strong women reflect a double rejection of the status quo—they're not just strong, but they are the gender who “shouldn’t” be strong. It’s no wonder strong women are so feared and so vilified, why I was made to be so afraid of them and made even more afraid of becoming a strong woman. If collective strength were to be oriented against power instead of in its support, there’s no telling what it might accomplish.

19

False Safety

OVER THE COURSE OF weeks, and then months, I worked my way up in the amount of weight I was squatting—65 pounds, 70, 80, 90, 100, 110. The reps came surprisingly easily. If I had just walked in the first day and loaded 95 pounds onto the bar, it would have Looney Tunes flattened me, leaving me painted on the ground. Yet here I was, the small amounts of added weight carrying me toward more and more power. I showed up to the gym, I put a little more weight onto the bar—an additional set of 2.5-pound plates, a new pair of 5-pound plates—and each time, on the whole, doing the reps and sets did not feel meaningfully more difficult than the last time. After the mechanical, unending struggle to burn more and more calories, this seemed like sorcery.

That was how it felt, at least, until the day I was set to squat 120 pounds. I loaded up the 45-pound barbell plus 37.5 pounds of plates on either side and started doing my reps. To the outside viewer, I moved as fast and smooth as ever. But I hesitated before the last rep, attempting to psych myself up. As I dropped down and rebounded out of the bottom of the squat, I psyched myself out, and hitched momentarily, like the space shuttle lost contact with ground control. The momentary neurological static threw me. I paused once upright, standing there in the rack, stunned, before reracking the barbell and ducking out from under it. What happened? Was it my form? What if I'd fully malfunctioned? I hadn't been even remotely prepared. Things had gone so well for so long that I'd virtually forgotten about even the possibility of failure.

I checked the weights to see if I had accidentally loaded more than I meant to, a mistake I made with some regularity—I hadn't. I began to wonder if the suddenness of the scare was metastasizing it in my head. Maybe it was just a blip and I was making too big a deal out of it. I passed my minute of rest time uneasily and then squared up to the bar, unracked, and completed my last five reps of 120 pounds as easily as I'd ever done.

During the next session a couple of days later, I loaded up 125 pounds. I unracked the bar and pumped out two reps. But on the third, my legs wobbled as if I'd been caught in a very local earthquake. I managed to stand up and then froze, holding the barbell on my back. I had two more reps to do, but already my body seemed to be giving out. Was this like last time? Was it worse? I couldn't quite remember.

I stood there, throttled with anxiety: and the longer I stood there, the more tired I was getting from just holding the weight on my back. I caved and reracked the bar. Now what? Did that count as a set? Could I have done those reps, and I was just psyching myself out again? Or—had I saved myself from certain grievous injury? What about my next two sets?

I turned from my barbell to the rest of the gym, and that's when I saw her: an actual other woman, setting up to squat on the other side of the room at Dimitrios's usual rack. (He was instead straddling a bench, cooler open, engaged in a midsession meal.) I'd felt sure I couldn't be the only woman who lifted at Richie's, but if there were others, we never seemed to actually overlap at the gym. Finally, we were in the same place at the same time, me and this other lady. She was short and thick, with two-toned hair done up in two braids, black on one side and creamy blonde on the other, with a few facial piercings and severely penciled eyebrows. She had loaded up some plates on the barbell—more than two hundred pounds—and was snapping on a thick leather belt with the word DEPTH embroidered on the back as she chatted with another guy in the gym. She turned from the conversation, ducked under the bar, and settled it on her shoulders before popping it up and out of the rack like it was nothing more than a broomstick. She squared her feet up and began pounding out her squats, one after another, until on her sixth rep, she juddered a bit. She didn't hesitate but continued right into the seventh rep as if nothing had happened. But as she came back up, her hips rose too fast and her knees shot inward, throwing her weight over her toes. She froze, trying to shift the bar back on track, but she couldn't make it happen—she slowly collapsed to the safety arms, which didn't stop the barbell from loudly clanging when it made contact. I winced. She was so short that I couldn't even see her down where she was probably pinned under the bar; I craned my neck trying to see over all the machines that separated us. But as I did, she popped back up, laughing as her friend slapped her on the back. She said something to him while she undid her belt, and he laughed, too. They started unloading the plates together so she could get the barbell back on the J-hooks.

I flushed with jealousy. I wanted that easy dynamic with anything I did, but especially with this thing that I had really grown to love. I had to face it: I was going to have to fail at lifting at some point, and I didn't feel ready for what might happen once I did.

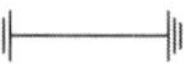

Failure in strength training has a specific technical meaning: when someone attempts a lift and then doesn't complete it for any reason, they "failed" it. It could be that their energy reserves were fully gone by the middle of the set, something distracted them and broke their focus, or they "misgrooved" the movement pattern of a lift and their muscles and nerves fired insufficiently or out of proportion or order. Or the challenge of a given weight was just too great, body parts gave out, and the weight fell to the ground, probably loudly.

Failure in lifting also has specific utility. Building strength is about pressing steadily upward on one's current limits. A lifter who fails occasionally, strategically, is making sure they are not undershooting their ability. Some of the most visible lifting content on social media is made up of elite lifters posting their personal-record attempts, usually from competitions. And they don't always succeed. Often as not, they or the weights, sometimes both, go crashing to the ground. They are often teetering on the razor edge between failure and, sometimes, world-record success.

So yes, online, I saw powerlifters fail their lifts all the time: spotters catching stacks of loaded plates as the lifters got stuck doing their squats, deadlifts that wouldn't budge, bench presses that collapsed on lifters' chests before spotters swept in to pluck them off. These lifters always bounced back and moved on to the next thing. "Not my best day," they might write in an Instagram caption. But years and hours and calories and technical expertise separated me from that. I had no spotters, no coach, no supporting crowd. I had Richie's Gym, a beat-up squat rack, a cookie-cutter starting strength program, and two legs that had been nearly evaporated by years of cardio, only just starting to come back.

For people who are new to lifting, failure is mostly what happens during the process of trying to find the sweet spot between "walk in the park" and "life-threatening exertion." But especially for unfamiliar beginners like me, this was a tricky line to draw. There is no ramp up or curve toward failure, and I understood it could happen erratically.

I normally and reasonably avoided failures of all kinds. But while lifting, I was expected to not only tolerate failure, but actively court it. *How will I know what "hard enough" versus "too hard" feels like?* I had to figure out how to fail, not just what it felt like to approach the line but what happened when I went over it.

Before watching my fellow woman fail just then, and aside from the random online failures, I couldn't recall having seen a single person fail at a lift in the gym, with the exception of bros doing "drop sets"—curling until their biceps gave out, in hopes that pushing over their limit would make their arms even bulgier. I'd already once drawn more attention than I wanted just by trying to do a deadlift; what would happen when I actually did something wrong?

Times like these, I would look longingly at the gym-machine forest behind me in the gym's mirrored walls. Even though Richie's machines all looked like they'd been chewed by a pack of wild dogs, they were inviting, with their cushioned seats and helpful diagrams and, most of all, the virtual impossibility of unpredictable failure. Still, I knew now they wouldn't give me what I wanted.

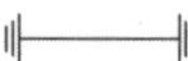

The book *Supertraining*, originally published in 1993 by Russian scientist Yuri Verkhoshansky and Mel Siff, PhD, is regarded in the modern strength-training space as something like the Bible, the urtext from which all other modern writings on strength training flow. In the book, the authors invented the concept of "block periodization." Rather than training the same way week in and week out, block periodization suggested that lifters would benefit from organizing their training into multiple specialized periods in order to better manage their energy: one for building up muscle size, one for capitalizing on the muscle size by building strength, and then a final block for concentrating that strength into new single-rep personal records. Now block periodization is the gold standard for how most people above a beginner level lift weights to get stronger, and it's one of the main reasons people are setting higher and higher records with much fewer injuries.

One of the topics *Supertraining* addressed was what the authors called "non-functional resistance" (NFR) machines—the machines that every chain gym, and even gyms like Richie's, pack into their square footage like herd animals. These machines first came onto the gym scene during the body-building heyday of the late 1960s and '70s and quickly insinuated themselves as the "high-tech," modern way to work out. But *Supertraining* argued the machines weren't worth the space they took up.

Before starting to lift, I had never realized there was a difference. I thought weights were weights were weights, and the choice of certain grunting individuals to use a squat rack instead of the quad extension machine was none of my business. Machines appeared more sophisticated and easier to use, and felt safer. They even had little instructional diagrams printed on them. Dumbbells and barbells, plates, and racks, on the other hand, came with no instructions.

But the slickness of the machines was exactly their problem. First, machines often require a person to work out each muscle individually, which is costly in terms of time. But Verkhoshansky wrote that machines are specifically counterproductive to what most people want out of the time and energy they put into fitness:

> NFR machines may be useful in concentrating more on the development of certain muscle groups for supplementing overall bodybuilding training or the primary stages of injury rehabilitation, but they are unsuitable for providing all-around conditioning of entire muscle groups…there is no single machine that can rival the training effect of a barbell squat, a barbell or a dumbbell curl, a barbell bench press, a power clean, a standing press, lateral raises with dumbbells or a barbell deadlift.

In fact, the authors said that the machines can be destructive to bodies:

> If a machine compels a user to use fewer joints and muscles than an equivalent free weights or pulley exercise, then the stress on all those structures will be increased proportionately. For example, the free standing squat involves three joints (hip, knee and ankle) whereas the seated knee extension machine constrains the body to use only one joint (the knee) in exercising the quadriceps, so that, in producing a comparable level of exercise over the same

> range of movement, this machine increases the shearing force across the knee. Moreover, the squat also offers the added advantages of exercising the thigh adductors, the spinal erectors, and several other stabilizing muscles, besides enhancing general balance and bone density...It is not often appreciated that seated exercise always imposes a greater load on the lumbar spinal discs than equivalent standing exercises...In the vast majority of cases, NFR machines provide an inferior, incomplete, and less efficient way of training the musculoskeletal system.

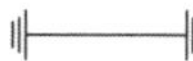

It was back to the muscles as a system again: gym machines wouldn't teach me to use my muscles in concert to stabilize and move me the way they were meant to, let alone teach me to use my body as I needed to use it in the real world. Even a machine that used multiple joints at once could take critical parts of the work away.

In bodies, the biggest muscles are often the "agonists" that perform the main action of the lift—glutes, hamstrings, quads. But in order to work, those muscles also need the "antagonist" muscles to chime in, as well as the "synergists." The same muscles can occupy different roles, depending on the movement. If I were to do a free-weight squat, the "agonist" glutes in my butt are being stretched and loaded up with tension, like a rubber band being pulled tight around the back of my hips as I lower myself down. They need my "antagonist" abs to oppose the movement and contract to keep my torso from falling forward, while the "synergists"—my quads on the front of my thighs, my adductors on the insides of my thighs, and my calves—help pace and control the movement. That's not all. My deep core muscles are also stabilizing me while I try to move the weight up and down, like the psoai that connect my lower back to the tops of my thigh bones, and my sartorii that connect the outside of my hips to the insides of my knees, and a bunch of other small muscles, ones too small for a machine to even target. That same squat with the weight set in a fully stabilized hydraulic track doesn't require nearly all of these muscles and would rob me of the stability I need to build up to handle that same weight in real life.

When it came to putting this into practice in the gym, based on that half set of shaky squats, I still hadn't built enough stability. I lowered the weight by a lot and finished my workout before going home, anticipating the next day when I would deal once again with what I considered, in many ways, the best but also most challenging part of lifting weights: resting.

20

The Secret of Doing Nothing

THE NEXT DAY I woke up hoping to let the beauty of rest wash over me. It was a Saturday in the summer, and as hot as ever. These were days when the city felt like a dryer full of wet clothes—they'd always been the worst days to run, and the heat and humidity never relented until after dark. I should have felt relieved to be off the hook.

I turned off the window air conditioner, hoping to save a little on my electric bill, and slid out of bed. I was out of the milk and yogurt I used to make my overnight oats, to which I'd become addicted over the last few years. I put on shorts and sandals and stepped out to make my way to the grocery store a few blocks away. The sidewalks were not yet radiating heat, but the sun was already glancing off shards of glass that littered the sidewalk from the nearby auto repair. Stripes of shade from intermittent tall buildings interrupted the blaze.

The grocery store was always freezing cold end to end, and I regretted not wearing a sweater. I sped through the aisles. In my earlier days in New York, with not a lot of money and a lot of nervous energy, I would pass the time by going on long walks in Manhattan, winding through the

Lower East Side, over to the West Village, up to Chelsea, over to Madison Square Park, down to the East Village, wearing holes through the thin rubber soles of my Target ballet flats. But per the strength-training doctrine, even walking qualified as cardio, which, the wisdom went, was a killer of gains—sapping too much energy away from my strength-training sessions could interrupt the flow of my progress. I could walk some, but I couldn't even cheat the system by logging my miles at a slower pace, even in the aisles of the grocery store. I would have to find my way to sitting my ass down.

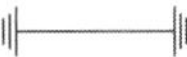

Before the late 1800s and the heyday of Muscular Christianity, the main enemies of bosses and lords and supervisors the world round were "idle" workers who willfully dawdled, who didn't have the same appreciation for the goals of their bosses—and didn't care enough about the good old Christian values of discipline and pleasing authority figures, including God. But the rise of the Industrial Revolution gave emerging productivity theorists a new golden template: the inexhaustible machines. Never mind a person's will to work; in competition with machines, they'd have no choice but to work hard all the time. But what about humans' sheer capacity? Could people be so reliably productive as machines in their work? Why did they tire out? As the hours of the workday dragged into the twelve-, thirteen-, fourteen-, fifteen-hour range, why did people's motions become sloppy, their eyes fogged, their brains thick? What if we thought of people as machines? And if we did, what if we could isolate and fix that which prevents them from just going and going and going forever?

During the Industrial Revolution, a meta-industry quickly rose up around the optimization of humans, and the race was on to extract energy from people like coal from a mine. Scientists created whole institutions dedicated to measuring and understanding the contours and limits of human energy. Academic journals filled up with publications of "ergonomic studies" trying to triangulate a relationship between factors of body weight, rhythm, heat, cold, anemia, and blood chemistry. Researchers tried to identify the essence of people of various races and ethnicities that led them to work differently—why did the Australian aboriginal, thought by the Europeans studying them to be inferior to Europeans, have a higher capacity for rigorous physical labor, while the effete Europeans swooned in the heat and became worn-out after much less time? Was it something in the blood, the brain, the skin, the sweat? (No one identified the likely real reason for "investigating" the difference: justification for subordinating native people.)

A German scientist, Wilhelm Reichardt, boldly attempted to develop a "fatigue vaccine" by experimenting with the blood of rats that he forced to exercise until they became exhausted and then eventually died. He claimed they died from a sharp rise in "kenotoxins" and then further claimed that he had developed an "antikenotoxin" with which humans could be injected, and that they would then be able to exercise for far longer than those who got a placebo. For good measure, in 1909, he tried spraying antikenotoxin into a Berlin classroom full of children, telling them the spray would improve the air quality. He then claimed that the students' "speed of calculations" increased by 50 percent, and that they made fewer errors. Other German scientists, excited by his findings, spent years retesting with their own experiments, only to find that Reichardt had badly exaggerated the effects of his alleged vaccine. The vaccine was followed by attempts to solve fatigue with more "nerve whips" like caffeine or cocaine, but they only delayed an eventual even worse collapse. There was no real trick to it, no hacking or manipulating the biological fact that people could not go and go forever. People were not machines. They needed some rest.

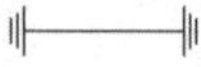

I had never had a relationship with the concept of rest. When I was a runner, days that I didn't run made me nervous. I waited them out uneasily, worrying about all the calories stagnating in my system and congealing into body fat. On days I couldn't run, I'd hold back even more than usual in eating foods. Days that I was supposed to run and then it rained, or snowed, or even tropical-stormed made me even more nervous. There was no telling what would happen if I couldn't follow my schedule; what if breaking my stride (literally and metaphorically) meant I never went back? I couldn't trust any lapse as anything other than a poorly concealed lack of will on my part; was the rain truly interruptive, or was I just using it as an excuse? What was I so afraid of—getting wet? Getting struck by lightning on one of the bridges crossing into Manhattan? Getting picked up by winds and dropped into the East River? I was tough; I could handle it, I told myself.

One of the earliest selling points of running to me had been the low barrier of entry, the fact that I could put on running shoes and step out the door and be achieving my workout anywhere. Over time, this became an obligation: there was nowhere I could hide, no sufficiently pressing excuse not to run. Everywhere, there was ground.

Often the rest days programmed in the free training spreadsheets for running I found online would be denoted as "rest day (or three easy miles)," "rest day (or cross-training)." I always chose not to skip a day if I could. In those programs, the authors seemed to be tacitly serving those of us who were propelled by a force that wanted nothing to do with reason and everything to do with continuing to go.

So for a while when I started to lift, I avoided my rest days and instead snuck in a furtive short jog on my Tuesdays and Thursdays. I couldn't make it more than three miles, thanks to my still-injured calves. But I couldn't just let all the cardio go; even though it had never worked to my satisfaction, I still couldn't be completely sure that it wasn't the only thing holding me together. I hadn't taken more than a few days off from running in years. But I was fighting the design of the program, and I suffered for it. I couldn't lift more weight each session, and I felt tired.

By this point, it was easy and intuitive for me to believe that working out (in a new and different way) would help me get stronger and that eating would help me get stronger. But resting *didn't* make intuitive sense because, frankly, I had never seen a workout program that involved so little working out. The training days already took only about half an hour. Then the recommended "rest" period between sessions was at least forty-eight hours, and as many as seventy-two. This gave the rest of a training week its structure around the three training days: one day on, one day off, and after three alternating days, two days off. Monday, Wednesday, and Friday to lift; Tuesday, Thursday, Saturday, and Sunday to rest. Four full days of rest and not working out...Put it this way: I had never even considered the idea of rest having its own intrinsic value, even in work.

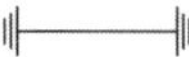

Exercise wasn't the only arena where I'd never given the value of rest a single thought. Years before Gamergate and my desire to cover it, I had started writing for that tech publication as a freelancer. I was afraid to make so much as a peep in the staff chat room. Every time I was assigned a story, I went into a virtual panic as I raced to finish it, turn it in, make my edits, and build it on the website as fast as I could. When the site gave me a part-time contract after a year and a half, I worked more hours than my contract covered, hoping to keep the editors at least satisfied. I had no idea where I stood until one day the editor in chief looked at me sideways at a rare staff happy-hour gathering in New York, after years of my near silence. "You know," he said, bemused but also clearly a bit in awe, "you never, ever complain." At first, I was totally unsure of what to make of this. The fact that the staff was distributed across the country and we had no real office meant I had virtually zero built-in visibility to everyone else's work interactions.

I learned eventually that all the other writers took far longer to complete their work, sometimes hours for a short post, to the annoyance of the editors. But everyone still had jobs at the website—real, full-time, salaried, benefitted jobs at that. It turned out the editors treasured how hard I worked and how I dedicated myself to whatever tasks they gave me. They didn't treasure my hustle with more money, of course, or health insurance, but with, you know, approval. Especially because I asked for nothing, ever, in return. I wouldn't have even known what to ask for.

As compulsive as I was at my work, lifting was about to teach me some difficult lessons. In my lifting program, rest days were not just "days that I didn't lift," or days when it was fine to actually do *some* activity, as long as it was less than the hardest days. Rest days, the blank days between the days with all the lifts and sets and reps written out, were expressly for *not* doing anything. The rest days were as important as the activity days. Having no rest days would negate all the hard effort of the activity days, and if I wanted the activity days to work, I had to take the rest days just as seriously.

The thing about muscles is that they are not actually built during workouts. When muscles move weights, their fibers get broken down and shredded up over the course of a workout. By the time a workout is over, the muscles have been damaged. Fortunately, bodies know exactly how to repair them: with time, nutrients, and most importantly, amino acids that come from protein. It's the repair process that rebuilds them to be better than before, and this is the crucial part of the cycle that actually creates new strength. Over time, the fibers become slightly larger, more interconnected by a nervous system that retains more learned reflexes from each practice session. And that isn't the only form of restoration. Muscles store energy in the form of glycogen made from sugar and carbs, and those stores get depleted over the course of a workout. Rest gives the muscles time to repackage and restock that fuel and be ready for the next session.

None of this repair can happen without time and space; a body that is still active and giving output can't manage its input. It needs both various forms of fuel to repair and time to use that fuel.

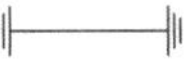

That wasn't all my muscles were doing on rest days, either. I had long been put off by lifting for a lot of reasons, but one of them had been the concept of calorie burning. I knew that burned calories meant weight lost. For all that grunting and sweating, if lifting burned only 200 calories per hour, on what planet would I voluntarily spend my time that way? What I didn't know then is that the world of exercise and calorie burning is far more nuanced than what any gym cardio machine alleges.

Obviously, calories aren't only burned during exercise. The process of burning calories while not working out is referred to in the science world as "non-exercise activity thermogenesis," or NEAT. It includes things like getting out of bed, opening doors, watering plants, brushing teeth, making dinner, picking socks up off the floor—anything that is physical movement but not truly purposeful exercise. NEAT accounts for between 15 and 30 percent of calories burned during the day and can vary by hundreds of calories between two people who are about the same size. But by at least one estimate, 72 percent of the difference in how many calories we burn just by existing (our "basal metabolic rate," in science terms) is down to how much lean mass we have. In other words, less muscle mass, lower NEAT. More muscle mass, though, higher NEAT.

One of my big problems was that, after years of dieting, my lean muscle, and therefore my metabolism and capacity for NEAT, had been absolutely thrashed. Because I had only been eating a tiny amount of food (for years), my muscle mass had been badly depleted, just in the course of trying to keep my body alive. This was why it felt like I couldn't eat very much without gaining weight. In part, my body was desperate to put pounds back on just because it needed calories and nutrients for all of its systems to function correctly. But it was also that I had effectively run through the little garden of my body with a torch. It seemed like it "held on" to calories because its ability to use calories and turn them into energy had been sabotaged.

It would be unfair to talk about these elements without noting that NEAT is influenced by a number of biological, genetic, and even environmental factors: for instance, someone who lives in a walkable area will trend higher for NEAT than someone whose city is designed for them to go everywhere by car. But to the extent that any individual can have their own meaningful effect on their metabolism, lean body mass in the form of muscle is one of the only levers there is to pull.

By eating more and working my muscles with heavy weights to trigger the rebuilding process, the cycle of damage I'd done over the last several years was essentially running in reverse: my muscle was being rebuilt, my metabolism was being restored, and I was burning more calories all of the time. I didn't need to be in constant motion to justify a (meager) caloric intake, because that had always been a symptom of a broken system and a reflection of my misunderstanding of what I needed. My body was still functioning at rest; it even needed the rest to rebuild my muscles.

So then of course I could *do nothing*. I'd done so well at doing everything else, but no one had even *seen* me try to do nothing yet. I would do the most nothing that anyone had ever done before! When I returned from the grocery store, I flumped down on my couch, and the cats arranged themselves around my legs as I pulled up an episode of *Veronica Mars*. I popped open a pint of peanut-butter-cup Ben & Jerry's, fighting to not care at all about the fact that, in truth, my minifridge had no real freezer to speak of. I'd eat my ice cream, I'd watch my show, I might even experiment with languidly falling asleep, huddled away from the summer heat.

After I'd eaten all the ice cream I could stomach, I put down the carton and huddled down on the couch. I closed my eyes and let the sound of Kristen Bell's voice wash over me. But my brain continued humming like an appliance. It was blissfully unconcerned that I needed to stop myself from wiggling around like an amoeba, or that if I could just sleep, I'd be seamlessly transported two, even three hours into the future. Hell, I wished I could wake up tomorrow, just in time for the gym. I opened my eyes to google "induce medical coma" on my phone, which surfaced a list of recreational drugs I was far too scared to take. I folded my arms over my chest and stared up at the ceiling. A million times, I had started workout programs and new diets, only for them to tail off after only a few days. This usually began with taking a day off. I knew all of the contours of treating myself like a deceitful degenerate, against whom I must maintain constant vigilance. The past wasn't perfect, but unlike this new future, it was entirely knowable.

With each new diet or workout program in the past, though, I had dreaded every new slog of a day: all the things I couldn't eat, all the tiresome rolling around on the floor doing leg lifts and chair dips. I actually liked proper lifting in the gym, much to my surprise. If I didn't and couldn't trust my whole self, I could trust that. I closed my eyes and drifted, finally, into a peaceful slumber. Two hours later, I awoke to half a pint of fully melted ice cream.

21

The Sandbox of Failure

KNOWING, AT LEAST THEORETICALLY, that failure was supposed to be a part of the lifting process, I wasn't about to give up on squats the first time they felt shaky. But this was the kind of hiccup that made me grateful for my rest days, because I didn't have to immediately face lifting again. I could pretend, for a day, that everything might go fine the next time, that the shakiness was nothing but a fluke. After a rest day, I returned to the gym for the first time to try again at 125 pounds. I squared up to the rack, one hand gripped on each side. Knowing that I'd come so close to failure the previous time, I felt sure this set was doomed, but I was less certain about what was still bothering me so much about failure.

Fear of failure for me was not about the failing itself—I knew that; I certainly *had* failed in the past. But every failure was painful to me. My early life had been filled with things I didn't know I was doing wrong until one or both parents were suddenly, fully in the throes of a meltdown: dad screaming at me for hitting a tennis ball against the garage door, mom crying because the forks were put away wrong. I couldn't predict these reactions, had no way to understand them except that I was the untrustworthy, unpredictable problem. Never mind the disaster scenarios where I had to hold myself just so and pray not to make things worse. This was echoed in all the ways I couldn't and shouldn't trust myself, with food, with rest. The wider world that equally didn't trust me, partners who didn't trust me, just reinforced what I already knew to be true. Actively courting failure, rather than working to avoid it at all costs, just seemed like pure, unbridled masochism.

The gym was so close I could exit my own door, blink, and be on the steps of Richie's. But I often extended the walk around a couple of blocks to warm up before my workouts, peering through the construction fences and into the foundation pit of a soon-to-come megasize luxury apartment building that would take up an entire block. Strangely, the area inside the fences was often devoid of activity, even in the middle of the day. I searched for workers or machines plugging away at their project, delaying my workout. As I tried to sit with my feelings about failure, I realized that those distrusting voices had become disembodied in my head but were always loud and at the ready, often manifesting as painful, irrational visual flashes of worst-case scenarios—the barbell crushing me, forcing my shin bones through my knees and severing my neck. I didn't just fear doing things wrong. I feared doing lots of things, at all: "wrong" being the always-possible outcome. I justified these feelings as a consequence: of being smart, having sense, taking on the work. Fear had become, in a backward way, the constant that I trusted.

This had made every step of the pulling-away process from my objectively horrible boyfriend wrenching (even through the silent looks of pity and confusion on my friends' faces). Breaking up with him was asking me to *dis*trust someone I wanted, badly, to love and trust precisely because I fundamentally didn't and couldn't love or trust myself.

I wanted desperately to have different instincts, different reflexive reactions to these kinds of situations, but they seemed to reach into my very biology, bad feelings rising like an atonal crescendo of an orchestra's largest and most ominous-sounding horn section. This conditioning made the biological background noise of my life one of extremes.

My familiarity with tension meant I was likely to overindex on perceived threats. My body was often on high alert: heart wanting to race, breath wanting to heave, blood pressure wanting to rise. And though I would panic fast, I always tried to manage the situation by freezing, presenting outwardly as if nothing were happening. I'd learned not only to ignore those biological signals of panic but to hide them, to see honoring them as the *opposite* of smart, safe behavior.

I had also come to feel that internal signs of calm—normal heart rate, breathing, blood pressure—meant that I was missing something, failing to index some threat. I had gone a long time almost incapable of feeling peace, not knowing what feeling peace meant, regardless of what was happening around me.

In her book *Trauma and Recovery*, psychiatrist Judith Herman breaks this type of response into three parts. First is the pattern of hyperarousal (the "persistent expectation of danger"), such that a traumatized person is always passively searching for threats. Then comes intrusion, the "indelible imprint of the traumatic moment," the constant presence of past traumatic moments as a filter for the present. This means that the traumatized person's threat search is heavily influenced by the events of the past, sometimes even on the lookout for signs unrelated to actual danger—for instance, they might experience rising panic in response to queues at coffee shops or theme-park rides, if one of their parents would react to those scenarios with violent anger or frustration. Lastly, there is constriction, the "numbing response of surrender," where bodies fight to detach from the moment as a protection against pain. When a person on constant watch for threats finds one (and they find them way too easily), they can respond by disconnecting from their bodies in anticipation of getting hurt.

So physical distress was, essentially, where I felt safe, in my own backward way: If threats were inevitable and I was experiencing them, at least I wasn't failing to perceive them. Dieting and cardio made twisted sense to me in a lot of ways, not least that they downregulated me, gave me a recreational venue for practicing that familiar denial of distress signals that

I'd learned as a little kid. They also gave the small relief of deadening the reflexes I kept tightly wound at all times. And when new outside sources promised me new ways to feel safe by self-denial, I was all too ready to listen. I lived in a soup of misguided reflexes and protective mechanisms that only self-reinforced.

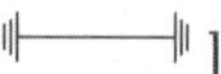

In elementary school, everyone learns the five senses: smell, sight, touch, taste, hearing. Sometimes these senses play a role in "grounding" exercises, which are often offered to people who struggle with anxiety or trauma. For instance, bringing yourself into the current moment by noticing five things you can see, four things you can hear, three things you can touch, two you can smell, and one you can taste.

We also learn in school that our bodies have processes that are voluntary and those that are automatic. We can't beat our heart on purpose, or process amino acids into muscle tissue or lipids into fat tissue. The gut biome processes food and the liver filters waste without us having to think about doing it. These are all governed by our parasympathetic nervous system ("para" from the Latin for "defend, protect against").

But there is a new emerging area of study in human biology on a separate set of senses that relate to our internal parasympathetic world. These allow us to perceive the metrics inside our seemingly coquettish, inconvenient meat sack: to hear or feel our heartbeat, our breath, tension in our muscles. This field is called "interoception," and the existence of interoception, or why and how some people seem not to have it, has been the subject of a deluge of recent research.

While we can swallow and breathe on command, sometimes feelings or events influence parasympathetic processes, and the effects spill over into the rest of our body. For instance, if we are jump-scared by a horror movie, our amygdala-driven reaction makes our heart rate spike and our muscles tense up before we have a chance to begin to feel anything emotional, or think anything intellectual, about the scare.

While there was a big uptick in the late 1800s of people diagnosed with neurasthenia (the popular but diffuse diagnosis for symptoms of fatigue, stress-related pain or cardiovascular issues, and depression), it faded out as a diagnosis before anyone could identify a consistent cause. But it shares many symptoms with what is now known as dysautonomia, or dysregulation of the autonomic nervous system that governs body functions like breathing, heart rate, and digestion. It also shares characteristics with chronic fatigue syndrome and fibromyalgia.

The research of Antonio Damasio at the University of Southern California in the 1990s found that when people with damage to their prefrontal cortex (the part of the brain that processes emotions and feelings) saw grisly or "emotionally charged" photos of, for instance, a car crash, they tended to have neither a physiological response as in the movie-watching scenario, nor an emotional response. These same people struggled with other higher-order tasks, like decision-making (the prefrontal cortex also handles executive functions like planning). Damasio suggested that perhaps all of these things are connected, that our ability to think clearly and make choices consistent with our values is related to our ability to attune and connect to our physical selves.

Evidence of the connection between our core physical self and our most sophisticated mental activity seems present in other groups of people facing health issues. People with depression have poorer-than-usual ability to sense their own heartbeat, which may be related to feelings of flatness and disconnection. Anxious people perceive changes in their heartbeats to be much bigger than they actually are, which could connect to their feelings of panic over relatively small challenges or changes. People with anorexia, one study found, have particularly poor interoception.

In the book *Overcoming Trauma Through Yoga*, the authors describe the way that dissociation, a way of compartmentalizing and distancing oneself from traumatic memories, can extend to the physical manifestation of pain: we learn from traumatic experiences to unplug from our bodies. But dissociation can lead to total fragmentation from our physical existence, turning bodies into an "other," or even an enemy, an inescapable foe whose onslaught of sensations and behaviors we've only ever known to betray us and make our lives worse. If bodily disconnection means that we are unable to recognize warning signs of pain and stress that our bodies are giving us, it also means we are unable to be truly present.

Still, just because two things are connected doesn't mean changing one will change the other. But like so many things that don't have a proven connection beyond correlation, scientists have experimented with using interoception to affect mental health. Various studies have attempted to regulate or soothe mental health issues by helping people better attune to their interoceptive signals. The results are limited but somewhat promising. One study of 121 anxious autistic adults found that three months of interoceptive training fully alleviated anxiety symptoms for 31 percent of the trainees, versus 16 percent whose symptoms were alleviated but received no training.

Another study posited that childhood trauma fosters a particular disregard for one's own biological signals. In the experiment, a group of 136 individuals with childhood trauma were evaluated for "interoceptive accuracy, sensibility, and awareness." The researchers found that subjects tested high for "body dissociation," or "the avoidance or disregard of internal bodily experiences and the feeling of separateness from one's own body."

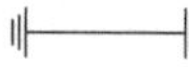

During the time I was growing up, neuroscientists considered brains to have a fairly straightforward and static developmental arc—they grow until they develop all the neurons they'll ever have, for better or for worse, at which point they begin their long, slow decline into old age. In the last couple of decades or so, an explosion of research has shown that brains are far more adaptable and capable of continued growth—or decline—throughout our lives than previously believed. They are capable of "neuroplasticity," altering or improving their function with the creation of new neurons (neurogenesis), increased brain-derived neurotrophic factor levels, and a few other processes.

The hippocampus is the part of the brain that forms and retrieves memories and also formulates emotional responses. People with post-traumatic stress (particularly chronic stress) and depression tend to have lower-than-usual hippocampal volume, due to both genetic and environmental factors. Another group with disrupted hippocampi? Disordered eaters. One study showed that people with anorexia nervosa had reduced hippocampus volume correlated with BMI, anxiety, and how hard the individual was striving to be thin; the authors specifically named malnutrition as a factor in lower hippocampal volume. A similar study showed that people with anorexia had lower hippocampal volume that was correlated with higher perceived stress. But when those anorexics recover, their hippocampal volume can recover.

In other words, food restriction can literally, biologically mess with the part of the brain that helps us incorporate new experiences into the fabric of our memories. Not only that—it can affect our emotional relationship to those memories, in the same way that trauma and other mental illnesses can. It was possible that food restriction had been part of what kept me trapped in accepting poor treatment and unable to process new validating experiences or people for what they were, distrusting them and treating them as threatening, the way I felt when I began to go to Richie's.

But scientists have also researched ways to stimulate neurogenesis in the hippocampus. It turns out that exercise is correlated with enhanced neurogenesis in this brain region, suggesting that exercise could be specifically healing to brain damage caused by trauma, stress, and too much dieting. Strength training, in particular, is correlated with improved cognition, and more recent research suggests this may be because it's also correlated with an increase in hippocampus volume.

The lifting lifestyle so far had already started to ease the chronic fear I had about many basic elements of life: eating, working out, resting, not dieting, getting stronger. I certainly cannot scientifically prove that gains were taking place in my hippocampus as well. Still, so much had been practically rehabilitated by breaking down my long-held rules. Failure was my specific hang-up, but among all the other ways lifting seemed to be helping my brain, this could be one more.

Now I longed to have a carefree and flexible sense of myself that could also withstand dropping a barbell, even once. A sense of self that wouldn't be triggered with anticipatory terror or waves of self-loathing. Unfortunately for me, comfort with dropping a barbell one time lay on the other side from where I was: having never dropped a barbell, even once.

Lifting, I saw now, was inviting me to see these failure situations as data: *this weight is too heavy; it's too soon to attempt this.* Could failing like this be a neutral experience that said little about me personally? Perhaps it could speak only to my relationship with the weights, to the fact that currently, things didn't work between us: a state that was no one's fault or shortcoming but simply revealed where I was situated in my strength journey.

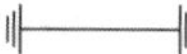

As I squared up to the squat rack for my doomed 125-pound set, I now felt sure this set was ordained by the swole gods to be a hard lesson in humility. A lesson in generosity to myself, in trusting the process, in accepting that progress would not always happen on my own perfectly comfortable terms. I looked at the fixed safety bars that extended resolutely to either of my sides, at about midthigh height. I'd never used them before for their proper purpose, which was to catch the barbell if I failed. I'd only lolled on them while I scrolled on my iPhone between sets. They were dented and dinged; I imagined the thousands who had come before me, who had attempted to squat similarly ambitious weights, only to collapse to the floor as the safeties stopped the falling barbell from crushing them.

I looked back at my reflection in the mirror, drew a deep breath, and ducked once again under the barbell. I aligned it on the backs of my shoulders, lifted it out of the rack, and started my descent. I breezed through the first two reps, though now I knew not to take this as any kind of promise. Mentally and physically bracing myself, I took a new breath and held it as

I dive-bombed into the third rep that had almost felled me before, and... stood up again, as if I'd done it a thousand times. What?

I stood there for a moment, stunned, before I took another breath and braced and dropped into the fourth rep. A little more effortful, but there I was standing once again. I lowered into the fifth rep and, with a little huff of effort, stood up as fast as I ever had. I walked the barbell back into the rack and looked again at my reflection quizzically. What had happened since my last attempt at this weight, which before I had barely managed, only to come back and perform my first set today as if I'd been born with 125 pounds on my back? I thrilled with confidence; maybe my faltering sets had all been a trick of the mind, a manifesting belief that I could only fail, was certain to fail, a blink in the staring contest of surety and resolve required by strength training. Maybe by *allowing* myself to fail in my mind, I had been *the very author of my unexpected success.* All I had to do, I thought smugly, was put my mind seriously to the task at hand, and victory would be mine.

Pleased with myself, I stepped under the barbell again and unracked it a second time. I pumped down into my first rep and rose unsteadily, faltering in a zigzagged line as I stood. Imperfect, but seasoned lifters like me were used to overcoming challenges such as these. All in a day's training! I sunk again into my second rep with the barbell on my back, but as I went to stand, I rose barely an inch before crashing the bar noisily onto the safeties, my body crumpling to the mat. Even against the throbbing bass of the rap music, the sound of metal on metal clanged throughout the gym.

I winced and squeezed my eyes shut, first at the sound, then in embarrassment. The barbell rolled away from where I was collapsed, purring as it went, to the end of the safety bars. This made room for me to stand, which I did slowly, my face hot in anticipation of all the indignant stares I knew I deserved for my noise, the racket of my hubris. But as I peeked discreetly around the room, not a single head was turned in my direction. The bodies continued to mill around and pump out their own reps, heads bobbing all out of sync, each to the beat of the music that played in their big, cushy over-ear headphones. I waited. Nothing. If I'd sneezed, I'd have gotten more of a reaction. I circled around to the side of the rack and began unloading the plates from the bar back onto the rack. Then I lifted the barbell off the safeties and back onto the rack for the next squatter. I pulled my notebook out of my gym bag, and where I'd written *125lb 3x5*. I wrote, *Failed second set. This was fine, actually!*

22

Body and Mind

BEFORE I'D STARTED LIFTING, I'd heard often of the "mind-body connection," but only in ways that annoyed me. When a yoga teacher asked me to extend my lower spine and root my bones into the earth, or "feel my shoulders in conversation with my hips"—what in the world?—at best, all I felt was a jumble of body parts that didn't seem able to do what they were already trying to do. *Get into warrior II pose, yada yada yada, feel your shoulders in conversation with your hips.*

Running, on the other hand, seemed to represent the mind-body thing at its worst. Its central conceit was getting to a level of sustained discomfort, even pain, and then disconnecting from my body in order to ignore it and transcend it. I seemed expected to be either in intimate, intuitive connection with myself, or denying and pushing myself away.

In lifting, the terminology was slightly different. Online coaches spoke of something called the "mind-muscle connection." With every rep, I was encouraged to dial in, consciously, to the muscles being called upon in that particular lift, directing mental energy toward them with the aim of getting physical energy to follow. It sounded, to be honest, very much like an internalized version of "the Force" from *Star Wars*, on a similar plane of silly fantasy. And in accordance with the *Star Wars* canon, my early attempts involved a rather strong effort straining to fight an invisible enemy, only to yield a big fat nothing and find myself abruptly exhausted and defeated. I would set up for a squat and turn my mind inward, directing it at my hips and glutes and hamstrings, and then begin the rep, trying to break down the neural walls to my posterior chain. I'd descend into the bottom of the squat and then back up, bouncing unsteadily off my knees and ankles, my lower back straining to heave the rest of my upper body back into position. I'd come back to standing, having failed to connect.

But occasionally, I felt a tiny glimmer of action; the rep would be slightly more controlled, less like falling through the air and more like a firing piston. I bounced less off my joints as my muscles started to respond and learned to slow me down and catch me as I fell. I looked up "activation exercises" online and tried them after my workouts were done. These were smaller, twitchier movements meant to isolate and build my connection with my glutes: clamshells, X-band walks, quadruped hip extensions. And one rep at a time, the connection built and built.

The thing about lifting weights that was different from other exercise related to the "mind-body connection" was that it had a language of progress. The *yada yada yada* that came before "feeling my shoulders in conversation with my hips," or whatever, was a matter of conscious practice and repetition, and the most important part was that it would not always or immediately be successful. It took time and consistent effort and, crucially, patience. Building connection, a steady and slow upward journey toward accessing various parts of myself, was the whole point. Just as people aren't born huge and muscular, strength training preached, they aren't necessarily born attuned to the interior parts of themselves. Even if I had a particularly warped or stunted connection with my body, I wasn't doomed to it forever.

In her book *Lifting Heavy Things*, somatic-experience practitioner Laura Khoudari writes about her experience helping her clients—some of whom are traumatized—reconnect with their bodies by lifting weights.

Where trauma causes people to disconnect from their bodies, conscious physical practice helps them learn to reconnect. This is referred to as "becoming embodied," which Khoudari describes as being "mindful of your body—its shape, weight, and density—and [having] the capacity to be aware of feelings and sensations that arise from it as and when they do (not after or before)." Because trauma causes disconnection from painful bodily experiences or sensations in hopes of surviving them, regaining this sensory capacity can be a tricky relationship to rebuild. But re-attuning to physicality and physical sensations can also become a bridge for re-attuning to many more abstract parts of the human existence: emotions, feelings of safety, trust, boundaries.

Before lifting, I had not once thought of myself, my body, as a mutable, habitable living thing. I had not even really thought of myself *as* my body. It was as if it had been a separate, unruly alien entity that I had to wrangle into submission, putting it through one obstacle course after another, wanting it to earn my approval, only to find it always falling short. (Often, the purpose of these entire exercises seemed to be setting the bar high enough that my body would always fall short.) I only allowed it to be useful as a vessel for tension, for the physical manifestations of dread and panic.

Every resource I read about lifting said that if I wanted strength, if I wanted to get back everything I had lost, I had no choice but to give my muscles my actual, undivided attention, if only for a few minutes at a time. Lifting forced me to be present in my body. I wasn't just a sack of meat for manipulating into the most pleasing shape; there was a whole world in there, nested layers of muscles and organs and sensations reaching out to my brain. My body was where I lived. Anywhere I might go in the entire world, there would be no escaping it. But fortunately, it was not the adversary I'd always believed it to be. Even after all this time, after all the neglect, after its decades-long depression nap, it was ready to wake up again. It had just been waiting for me to see it.

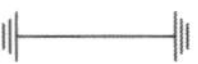

Interoception and embodiment may explain why physical activity, and especially strength training, has the potential to help people who have experienced trauma. Trauma interrupts interoception and disconnects consciousness from our bodies, through dissociation (feeling markedly disconnected from the world around us) or depersonalization (having a feeling that we are observing ourselves from outside our bodies, that the world around us is not real, or both). This happens in moments of acute trauma, but these are also feelings that can persist in a chronic way throughout our lives, for people, for instance, with forms of PTSD. People with PTSD are also more likely to suffer from conditions like chronic pain, which further alienates them from themselves.

Embodiment could be fundamentally important for re-attuning to our interoception, developing a sense of self, and regulating emotions. This is because sensing our bodies, our physiological reactions, is critical in attuning to our feelings. Good perception of the physical signals of having a feeling may be key to good perception of the emotion itself. In that way, lifting became not just about developing muscles for me; it became about developing feeling, developing my literal sense of myself. Instead of ignoring and pushing down my body's signals, I was learning to both hear and trust them as a source of important information.

In *Trauma and Recovery*, Herman writes about the importance of empowerment in rehabilitating from trauma, especially in developing autonomy and "engaging more actively in the world" as a counter to feelings of helplessness and isolation. Specifically, Herman cites "a conscious choice to face danger" as a kind of controlled sandbox for developing new responses and "rebuild[ing] the 'action system' that was shattered and fragmented by trauma." As a result of experimenting with danger, survivors "may begin to question previous assumptions…Women question their traditional acceptance of a subordinate role. Men question their traditional complicity in a hierarchy of dominance." Lifting was, perhaps, the danger sandbox that I needed: controlled but unfamiliar. Challenging and uncomfortable, but tolerable. Most of all, it was easily scalable to my level: Thirty pounds too heavy? Twenty will do.

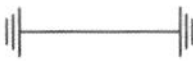

The danger sandbox that is useful for unlearning the physical aspect of trauma also comes up in experimenting with pain. Fear of pain and discomfort is a huge deterrent for many people in physical training, and those who haven't had time or space to experience a "safe" amount of pain can understandably be alarmed by any pain. My siblings and I, competitive as we were, spent all of our young years dancing around this line, wrestling, fighting, playing sports, falling from and being pushed off of play structures or trees. I have, essentially, a field PhD in pain. Not everyone is so lucky. It does not help that, for many years, the practice of working out was almost inextricable from slogans like "no pain, no gain," "sweat is your fat crying," and other maxims conveying that more intensity and ignorance of pain are always good things. This messaging not only overrode what should be a valid concern about pain, but it also didn't allow for a framework where people could develop a relationship with pain other than "pain is both terrible and needs to be maximized." Pain can be good, especially when a little managed pain now can prevent significant unmanageable pain down the road. When we open up the experience of pain from the rigid maxim of "the less pain, the better," there are many greater possibilities for our relationship with pain.

What we might call "practice with pain" doesn't simply reduce the specter of pain as something to fear, or the actual sensations of pain; it can give us a more expansive and dimensional relationship with risk in general. Pain is a spectrum like many other things, and our relationship with it is capable of development and change. For the times when unavoidable pain (emotional, physical, metaphorical) does happen in an uncontrollable way, we can be much better prepared to handle it with this kind of foundation.

In a 2015 study cited in the book *Ouch! Why Pain Hurts, and Why It Doesn't Have To*, children who were allowed to engage in risky play for a fourteen-week period showed greater "self-esteem, risk detection, competence and a decrease in conflict sensitivity." When kids aren't able to establish a relationship of agency with pain—that it can be a continuous and survivable negotiation in which they have a say—they are "more likely to develop problematic behaviors around hazards, phobias and overwhelming fears."

For those who deal with too much unpredictable pain, it can lead to pain "catastrophizing," which prompts our bodies to overstate, to the brain, the amount of pain they are experiencing. But being too accustomed to pain can also be a bad thing: people who are overly "habituated" to pain will tend not to take pain as a signal to modulate what they are doing until it's too late, resulting in injury. Predictably, people with less interoceptive ability need more practice at dialing back in their activity based on how much pain they are experiencing.

Pain is an inevitability for anyone training with any degree of ambition—even, say, a young woman attempting to squat 125 pounds for the first time. Elite athletes, specifically, the authors of *Ouch!* write, are extremely experienced at negotiating their relationships to pain. "Pain is not something that just happens to them; they have a say in what it means, in how it is experienced in the present and remembered in the future," the authors write. "Athletes don't just ignore pain and push past it. They assess it and reframe it. They've learned how to negotiate with pain…They take control." Or, turning this on its head: athletics (including training, or even just regular exercise) give people a realm in which to sandbox our experience with pain.

In the study of rehabilitating our relationship with pain on a mental and emotional level, people with arthritis are some of the most popular subjects, in part because we can be sure their pain is not going away, but also because living their lives to any degree necessarily involves interfacing with pain. For people with arthritis, life is pain, not in the metaphorical or romantic way we sometimes say that, but in a literal way. And the only choices on the table are whether and how to manage that experience.

Until recently, the interventions for arthritis were almost exclusively medical, focused on mitigating the physical fact of pain. But in a 2006 research review, occupational therapist Dr. Catherine Backman looked broadly at what happened when people with arthritis received treatment for the "psychosocial" aspects, from experiencing anxiety and helplessness to maintaining leisure activities. The treatments Backman looked at included coping skills as well as cognitive behavioral therapy. Across the board, rehabilitating their relationship with pain not only decreased anxiety and depression related to the pain, but helped reduce the pain itself, "at least in the short term," Backman wrote.

Studies about the inevitability of or need for pain aside, we often have specific prejudices about exercise-related pain. Popular discussions around pain and athleticism often focus on elites setting world records who are pushing through blinding pain, which can reinforce our perception that exercise is only worthwhile if it involves as much pain as possible.

In fact, I was finding that as the results of my training steadily built up, workouts with no pain, or a small amount of pain, were far from meaningless. "Gain" does not increase as "pain" increases. There is no valid strength-training program in the world that measures progress in terms of pain. Though my strength had multiplied many times over the course of several months, I had not once suffered beyond some mild soreness. In truth, I'd suffered more in the past from "core workouts" printed in the backs of magazines, attacking my midsection with thirty minutes of crunches and planks that stressed my muscles out so badly I couldn't laugh without pain the next day. I hadn't known at the time that steady progression, as well as recovery—rest, and especially food—plays a huge role in mitigating post-workout pain and soreness. Once I started eating, particularly, it eliminated that dreaded aspect of training that I'd previously grimly accepted as inevitable.

I did not always nail it. Many times, I didn't eat enough following a workout, only to wake up more stiff and sore than usual the next day. Eating more that day helped, but it was mostly a reminder to be serious about eating the next time. The early days of lifting were a swift upward trajectory, but as time went on and I took some time off, that meant I had to restart working out. I'd be tempted to jump in where I'd left off. Once, after more than a month off, I returned to the gym to work out and ambitiously loaded up 155 pounds on the barbell. Midsquat on the second set, my legs cramped up so hard I couldn't finish. The next day, I was unable to even sit down on the toilet.

After that incident, I started to cherish the window of "getting back into it" as one where it was virtually impossible to take things too easy. If I'd been squatting two hundred pounds before the break, I'd start with sixty-five pounds when I resumed. Being comfortable with pain was one thing, but actively courting unnecessary pain was another. Life was going to hurt anyway; if I could use what I knew to avoid it, I would.

In the grander scheme, the slow awakening of my muscles didn't just show me that I could get stronger. Lifting was the sandbox where failure could safely happen and mean nothing about my life in the bigger picture. I'd become so tightly wound that putting a single toe out of line, at work, while eating, had felt like a dangerous idea. Now, danger was becoming survivable, and time spent fearing it was a waste.

Part Three

As I hoisted my own luggage into the trunk, my very Polish cab driver, impressed, shouted "STRONG GIRL!! FARM??" And this is the only way I wish strange men to speak with me moving forward.

—@TrinAndTonic, on X

23

Being Watched

ONE SUNNY DAY, AFTER several months of faithfully posting up at Richie's to lift, I arrived in the gym at lunchtime to squeeze in a workout. At this time of day, it was sparsely populated; there weren't more than a couple people on the cardio machines, a few winding their way through the weight machines, and a handful scattered along the back wall using the dumbbells. It usually got more crowded as the afternoon went on. Both squat racks were open, so I grabbed the one closest to the center of the room. My earbuds were already in, and I was listening to "I Wanna Dance with Somebody" by Whitney Houston. I began to warm up, first with just the barbell, then adding my small plates every set. But after my second set, I noticed some motion out of the corner of my eye. I turned, and there was a man hanging off one of the nearer machines, gaze studiously fixed on the ground, partly obscured by long, greasy-looking hair and a black baseball cap. He fiddled with the equipment with one hand and was holding his smartphone in the other.

I turned back to what I was doing, but as I unracked the bar and set up to start squatting again, I saw motion again, maybe a reflective flash of light of the kind that didn't normally come from the dimly lit center of the gym. I turned, and the man was now holding his phone to his ear, as if he were having a conversation. The glossy back of his phone glinted. I turned back to center and returned to doing my warm-up squats. On the third rep, again I saw a visual artifact out of the corner of my eye. At the top of my squat, I stopped and turned my head to look, and I saw the man raising the phone, just barely too slowly, back up to his ear. As he did, he pivoted his head away from my direction to gaze intently up at the ceiling, as if he'd lost something up there. He'd been filming me. He had been standing in broad daylight, pointing his smartphone camera at me, and recording. I wasn't close enough to see his phone screen to know, but I knew.

I turned back and reracked the bar, ducked out from under it, and stood there again, facing my reflection. I'd had an incredibly good run at the gym. Until this moment, basically every nightmare scenario I'd had about feeling unwelcome or alienated or objectified hadn't come to pass. The psychedelic anxiety I'd felt about interacting with this world had virtually dissipated. But now here I was, and here he was, reducing everything I'd fought to feel okay about into some pixelated little video that he was going to do God knows what with.

I felt the swirl and pound of my body's alarm system, breath, pulse, nerves, reaching from the pit of my stomach into my throat. The simple reality of it wasn't even the worst part. What if this had happened before, had long been happening, had *always* been happening, in one form or another, with other people in other situations, and I'd failed to notice? The only thing worse than it happening once was it happening for a long, ongoing time in a pervasive way, due to my false sense of security, my hubris, my stupidity. But this time, I was determined not to disconnect. I would not, I resolved, black out from terror at this guy who couldn't just watch internet porn like normal people.

I couldn't be 100 percent sure the guy in the gym was filming me. But the signs were there. I had to trust my judgment. He wasn't going to take this from me. I looked around for help. Dimitrios was off in the far corner of the gym heaving some of the largest dumbbells Richie's had to offer, but he didn't seem like the right person to bother.

I turned from the squat rack and headed toward the front desk, a path that would have taken me past the filmer if he hadn't virtually barrel-rolled away into the weight-machine forest. I rounded the corner and stepped up to the desk attendant, who looked up at me.

"Um, I'm not sure really what to do here," I said to him, "but I think this guy has been filming me."

"Which one?"

"He's over there—black hat. He was pointing his phone camera at me like this." I pointed mine at him as if I were filming him.

The attendant fixed his gaze just below the counter and began clicking on a mouse and keyboard. These counters always looked simply like counters, and I forgot that they were there in part to conceal monitors fed by cameras that, in this case, surveilled every corner of the gym.

"Where were you?"

"Over at the squat rack closest to us."

As the attendant reviewed the monitors, a second employee behind him jumped into action and swooped from behind the desk to go get eyes on the guy. Shortly, he returned. "Yeah," he confirmed. "I can see him watching the video."

The first attendant, satisfied by this report and what he was able to see on the monitors, picked up a phone and dialed a number, stepping away and into the rest of the gym. When he reappeared, he menacingly herded the guy in the black baseball cap, eyes on the floor, out the front door.

As the attendant returned inside, he came back up to me. "He's banned for life," he told me. "I told him to delete the video, but who knows? Someone else stopped me to say they'd seen him, like, on the subway, filming women like that," he said.

"Wow," I said. It all happened so quickly. "Thank you for...being so on top of it." I had been steeling myself for not even so much as a "yeah, we'll look into it" when I approached the desk. Instead, these two young guys had gone full SWAT mode (perhaps not even out of a sense of justice so much as finally getting a break from the sheer tedium of a job that otherwise consisted of clocking members in and out of the gym and restocking paper towels). Still, I was impressed.

"Yeah. Let us know any time if it happens again," said the second attendant. "We don't want people like that here."

Dimitrios appeared at the desk. "What happen?" he said. "Someone bother you?" He looked me in the eyes and held up a fist. "We get him out! You tell me! I fix straightaway. No bullshit. You tell me."

I thanked the guys at the desk again and walked away a little unsteadily. I was still shaken at having my delicate little bubble pierced by this weirdo. But just as quickly as it had happened, the gym had redeemed itself and then some. And I'd gone from feeling like I might finally be chewed up in exactly all the ways I'd always feared only to find that more than one person was willing to help me wedge the jaws open.

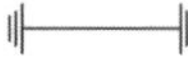

Unlike the supportive environment I was realizing I'd found at Richie's, I'd recently recognized the opposite about my day job. Several days after the iCloud leak of celebrities' nudes, I wrote a follow-up article on Gamergate and gave it to an editor whom I didn't usually work with. He edited it indifferently, suggested I remove a paragraph I thought was essential to the perspective of the story, and directed me to go ahead and publish it. I left the paragraph in and posted it.

A short time later, he blew up at me in direct messages, accusing me of undermining his authority. I told him I'd misunderstood what I thought was a suggestion but that he'd apparently meant as an order. His undertone, though, was that this was about more than disobedience; the paragraph represented an overstep from the "objectivity" that I was supposed to (selectively) apply to articles about gender politics. It couldn't even be, just maybe, that I was right; it could only be intentional defiance.

By this time, I'd worked there for five years, but after all that time, how little I'd complained didn't matter, not when it came to arguing against something as relatively straightforward as people who had been hacked, women who had been doxed. The people I worked with preferred to do whatever it took to remain in the good graces of guys who seemed like they'd call in a nuclear strike on a female game developer's house if it protected the polygonal boobs with pointy nipples in *Grand Theft Auto*. The irony would have been painful if it weren't so laughable.

A few weeks later, I called up the editor in chief to say that I was quitting.

"Well, you're not very good at your job anyway" was his response.

After I hung up the phone, I stormed around the corner into the gym. I was intent not on squatting or bench-pressing the barbell so much as fighting it, throwing every ounce of anger and injustice I felt into moving the weight. My early sets moved easily, so I loaded on ten pounds more than usual. Music pounded in my earbuds as I panted in between my sets. I loaded on still more weight; I wanted to fly right at the ceiling of my strength. I no longer feared it, was no longer tiptoeing around lest it collapse on top of me. Now I was hunting it like an animal, daring my strength to show itself. Before I knew it, I was fighting through reps with thirty more pounds loaded on the bar than usual. My legs virtually knocked knees as they quivered through the last rep, my face red. After I stood up, I slammed the bar back into the rack and unwrapped my shoulders, stood hanging my arms from it, head drooped in between.

For weeks, I'd feared continuing to push up in weight, completing each set more and more warily, dreading the failure I knew would be coming my way. And yet here I was, having launched myself into what felt like a stratospheric amount of weight to squat, ever, let alone for multiple reps. I was mad at my editors; the only thing more pathetic than being a Gamergater was being afraid of them. But I was also mad at myself. I'd worked my ass literally to the bone for approval according to those values, without really stopping to consider what that approval meant. The moment I stopped, not out of malice or some chaotic impulse but just to stand up for something I believed in, one time, all that approval had turned out to be conditional.

Still, what I would have normally done would've been to push everything down and give in, and the tension of doing one thing but feeling another would have boiled within me. I would have been restless, awake through the night, alert, miserable, acutely aware something was wrong but unable to identify or honor exactly what it was. Even as I was in the gym hurricaning my body around, there was an eye to the storm that felt clear.

I stepped back from the barbell, unlatched my thick leather lifting belt, and picked up my phone to text my former coworker—now soon-to-be boss at the job I'd lined up—about what the editor in chief had said to me. Her agreement that he was being a jerk flooded into my jacked-up nervous system, quenching its many electrical fires. I also found a text from my friend Hannah: *I want to try lifting weights. Will you show me?*

Of course, I wrote back.

By this time, I was talking about lifting to my friends constantly; some had been infected by my rabid enthusiasm for lifting and told me they were eager to try it. I'd bring them to the gym and show them the ropes, and while they were also a little disbelieving that the workouts could be so short, they liked that it wasn't a slog. Mostly, they seemed apprehensive of approaching the weights by themselves and wanted a metaphorical muscle, as well as someone with literal muscles to help them feel like they weren't in someone else's way. Just like my experience, when I brought them to Richie's, almost everyone was unfazed by their presence.

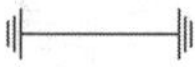

When I reached out to schedule a date to go to the gym, Hannah told me more about her workout journey. She'd become disillusioned with her most recent attempt at getting into a routine, with a program that involved way more humiliating jumping and bouncing around than she felt comfortable doing in her crowded gym, and she felt hungry all of the time. The program was called the Bikini Body Guide by Kayla Itsines, a series of lengthy high-intensity workouts and a punishingly restrictive meal plan, PDFs of which were furtively traded around online. Itsines marketed the program by posting young girls' midriffs over and over on Instagram, the skinny "before" on the left and the emaciated "after" on the right.

Itsines's content was part of the dark side of fitness social media I had been less aware of during its early days of 2011 and 2012, when the platforms were a Wild West with less regulation and oversight than would be imposed on them over the next decade. Social media posts already had the power to stir insecurities and feelings of comparison and inadequacy. Some posters quickly capitalized on this, bringing in brain-worm memes like the "before-and-after" picture and posting them to a place where no one was checking whether they were making the "results not typical" disclaimers that were required of TV and magazine ads.

Once the curation algorithms came to social media in 2016 and supplanted the chronological feed, they magnified the insecurity effect, bubbling up posts that fed compulsive, sweaty, constant use. Quick health fixes and workout programs promising the world threaded the needle of "attractive premise + barely plausible spellbinding solution." They kept people swiping—workout routines to get abs in two weeks, a particular supplement that supposedly fueled a higher metabolism. The closer the content skirted the line of "barely plausible," the more viral it seemed to go: "nature's breakfast cereal" that was just berries in a bowl of ice water, "increasing cognitive abilities" by consuming antifungal dye meant for cleaning fish tanks, "blood flow restriction bands" to tie around limbs that purported to make workouts more effective. At a different time in my life, I would have been sucked in hard by this world.

The Bikini Body Guide was later absorbed into Itsines's subscription mobile app, Sweat, which she sold in 2021 for $150 million. Years later, many followers of Kayla Itsines claimed her client testimonials on Instagram triggered, hastened, and worsened the onset of their eating disorders and body dysmorphia, damaging their physical and mental health and sending some of them to treatment.

As quickly as the earnest online world that made lifting possible for me appeared, it vanished again, like a brief, shimmering dimensional rift. The women I'd loved for just sharing their lifting journeys were replaced with people boosted by the algorithms shouting into the camera, "Here's your reminder," "I just need people to know that…," "What they don't want you to know is…"—baby-food content they were trying to airplane into my mouth. One by one, the accounts I followed either transformed into something unrecognizable in service to the algorithm, with the steadily vaulting follower and engagement numbers to prove it, or their posts slowed to a trickle before drying up completely. The algorithm couldn't understand the pricelessness of their unpolished, unpuréed enthusiasm, so even if they still existed, it buried them.

24

The Beauty of a Good Bulk

DURING THE FIRST TWO years I was lifting, I got far stronger than I ever imagined I would. With practice, all the moving parts of my new habits got easier and easier to sync up: eating, feeling comfortable in the gym, failing, tinkering with my form. I started walking into the gym as if it were my second living room (well, my only living room, since the living room in my apartment was actually an office, bedroom, and kitchen). Some of my fears had come to pass: getting pestered by the personal trainer, being sexually harassed by the creepy filmer. But lifting was simply too fun, too gratifying, and made me feel too good to cede it to a couple of losers. And more importantly, they had proven to be the rare and unwelcome exceptions within the gym (and I never saw either of them again). Meanwhile, everything I'd dreamed of—working out a normal amount, no longer experiencing cravings, eating a regular amount of food—had happened.

Lifting had laid bare the lies I'd been told about how food and bodies worked. I didn't have to scrape by on 1,200 calories a day, praying not to gain any weight. With a little additional muscle, my metabolism could easily take care of far more than 2,000 calories a day. My body could feel good to be in, powerful even, instead of like an increasingly rickety abandoned building.

Still, after all this time, the gains train had started to slow down. I was still eating a lot and lifting a lot of weight, but the amount of weight I was lifting was not going up as reliably as before. When I tried to squat 185 pounds, it made my legs quiver. I backed down the weight to check my form, but when I went back up, my muscles trembled like wet Chihuahuas. In fact, all the lifts began to feel hard in a way I wasn't used to. I struggled, sweat, and strained as my elbows drunkenly wandered this way and that during bench. My back hadn't been straight during a deadlift in weeks. I was failing my lifts, and not in a "mistakes are how we grow" way.

I'd seen a bunch of my lifting heroes do this thing when they wanted to get stronger: they ate extra to get extra energy in the gym, which let them train harder, which made their muscles grow, so they needed to eat even more. It was called "bulking."

Bulking is one of the less-understood parts of gaining strength in the wider world, in part because it is instantly counterintuitive to the "weight loss = good" principle. Bulking is the term for when lifters intentionally *gain* weight, with the purpose of getting stronger. It's not as simple as just eating a lot, *yada yada yada*, you get stronger. But it is not wildly more complicated than that, either.

We are all taught what happens when we eat more calories than our body can use: The extra fuel gets stored, mostly as fat under our skin or around our organs. But this is not the only possible outcome. The difference depends on what our bodies are doing as they are receiving these extra calories.

When we eat extra (often called a "surplus" during a bulk), not only do those calories give us extra energy during strength-training sessions, but they make it possible to cause more muscle damage than usual. And that extra fuel and protein don't just fuel a hyperpowered session; they fuel an extra-intensive recovery, particularly once the easy recomposition days are over. This means muscle can still grow and we can continue to get stronger. Instead of the caloric surplus adding only body fat, it adds muscle too.

I ran the numbers on how much I'd have to eat: My maintenance food intake was 2,300 calories. The strategy I was going to try required adding 20 percent on top of that, which came out to 2,760 calories. In real terms, that was not so much more food; it was equal to an extra good-size bowl of ice cream every night.

Eating an extra almost 500 calories each day meant I'd be eating nearly 3,500 extra calories per week, which worked out to exactly one pound of added body weight per week. According to my trusty sports dieting book, *Renaissance Woman*, I could expect about half of that to be muscle, maybe slightly more if I was lucky. If I bulked for three months, that meant I'd only be gaining twelve pounds—six pounds of muscle and six pounds of fat. For most of my life, these numbers had been normal scale fluctuations—much less of an impact than I might have guessed would come from a "bulk."

The math of it was reassuring; whether I'd stick to the math was another question. If I started a bulk, I'd be forced to finally confront my longtime body fear: becoming "bulky."

My size had always seemed to stay the same when I had been eating very little, and that made it seem like it might skyrocket when I started eating more. But as I'd seen over the last couple of years, it hadn't happened, especially once I'd built my muscle back. When I started lifting, I also started eating about 50 percent more, and I was still wearing all the same clothes.

I already loved eating a lot, and loved lifting even more, so the idea of eating more to lift more was not exactly a hard sell. I had reached a new understanding of my body, of all the positive feedback loops that came from eating and training and resting. My body could do things, including get stronger; it wasn't just ornamental, or just a jar to carry my brain around. But I had never deliberately gained weight before in my entire life. I had gained weight before by accident, and so tenuous was my sense of self that those twenty pounds had knocked me out of orbit and careening deep into the black of disordered space. From that time on, I had organized all of my life around not gaining weight—and continuing to attempt to lose weight, just in case I was gaining it and somehow not realizing it.

I wanted to be enlightened enough to gain weight dispassionately, but a part of me hadn't really changed. How could I be sure that, once the floodgates of eating were fully open, I wouldn't turn into a bottomless pit? What if I threw the careful new orbit I'd found off its axis, and bulking became a pretense for just eating endlessly? What if I destroyed the beautiful equilibrium I'd finally found?

The problem was that I loved training. I wanted to be stronger. I was sick of struggling with my bench press; I wanted to do a pull-up; I wanted deadlifts to finally click; I wanted my squat numbers to keep going up. If gaining weight was all that it took, I owed it to myself to try it.

Because my program had stopped yielding the forward progress I wanted, I toyed around with a few new options before landing on one that integrated strength-focused sets along with hypertrophy-focused sets of six to twelve reps. "Hypertrophy" is the fancy term for "muscles get big." A fixture of the strength world, Greg Nuckols, had theorized on his much-trafficked website Stronger by Science that "powerlifters should train more like bodybuilders." Nuckols pointed out that big people weren't necessarily strong, and many strong people were not very big at all. But for most of us in the middle of the talent road, strength tended to trend upward with size, revealing a positive feedback loop between the two.

While size didn't necessarily produce strength, it created bigger muscles that could then be recruited to the purpose of strength, and more strength was what I was after. "A bigger muscle, all other things being equal…, is a stronger muscle. There's no way around it—past a point, you simply have to grow," he wrote. This meant that not only was I confronting gaining weight, I was confronting getting bigger and more muscular, too.

I set a date for my bulk to end in three months and began digging in. I added eggnog to my breakfast overnight oats and extra noodles to my

Bolognese, and I piled the Parmesan high; I added Oreos and Hershey's syrup to the blender for my protein shake, more ice cream, more snacks. Juice, chips, bread and butter—all the things I'd long avoided became priority number one if I wanted to get all my calories in by the end of the day. I used a kitchen scale to be sure of the amounts.

I had worried I might start inhaling every food in sight. If anything, I had the opposite problem. In practice, eating enough to bulk, every single day, was not as easy as it seemed. One day, I mistakenly ate a too-light meal as I ran from a meeting to a PR event, with time only to grab some bodega packages of nuts and chips instead of a proper lunch. As I pieced together my foods eaten so far in the food-tracking app, it handed me a 2,000-calorie deficit. No problem, I figured; this is what McDonald's is designed for. I started plugging in McDonald's foods, one after the other, until I had a meal that brought my calories to where they needed to be: a Quarter Pounder with cheese, a McChicken sandwich, a large fry, and a medium chocolate shake. And I'd have to eat every last bite, leaving only crinkly wrappers behind. My days of WeightWatchers-inflected dieting had taught me that young ladies who wish to keep the pounds from piling up should eat their food slowly and carefully, savoring and thoroughly chewing each bite, in order to feel their fullness. But as I sat down to my McDonald's feast, I cast off the chains and I ate as quickly as I could, alternating sips of shake and bites of food like I'd seen competitive eaters do on TV.

The idea that if I began to want, I might never stop was a lie I'd been told about myself for so long that it had become one of my core beliefs. But what I discovered when I started eating for lifting was that my cravings and food fixations were simply a product of the deprivation I'd undergone. Once I gave myself basic sustenance, it turned out I was not some insatiable maw, a needy black hole of unquenchable desire. I was a human alive on Earth; I needed some goddamn food. Bulking turned out to be the same: throwing open the doors to even more food didn't change anything. I weighed myself on my former enemy, the scale, to track my weight to make sure I was eating enough. The number jumped all over the place for a while, but after a few weeks, it formed a smooth upward trendline.

In working out for strength, I'd become attuned to my body in a new way. Working at the outer limit of my capacity for intensity had slowly grown my awareness of my energy, how I was feeling. Drinking an extra beer or going to bed too late wouldn't affect the way I'd go for a walk. But in lifting, the fatigue or stress could sometimes jump out mid-bench or mid–squat session, making me realize that I did, in fact, perhaps go too far the previous night ordering a round of tequila shots. This and a million other things could affect working-out energy, so I learned not to be too attached to "being in the mood" or "feeling like it"; a middling day, energy-wise, was plenty to keep me moving forward, and I didn't actually have to be at 100 percent every session to keep building. Even days that I felt the least like lifting were usually the days I was the happiest I went and did it after all—80 percent, or even 60 percent, was better than nothing.

The thing about bulking, though, was that it produced the opposite feeling of too many tequila shots. Maybe it was because my body had been in a kind of nuclear winter for so long, but when I arrived in the gym the first time all stacked with extra carbs, I felt like a live wire. I pulled up to the squat rack absolutely crackling with energy. Oftentimes, the warm-up sets I'd do before I actually began my workout were a process of shaking myself awake and reaching pace, like swimming through seaweed to get to clear water. Now, I was rampaging through them as if on a Jet Ski. Reps that I had struggled with the previous week flew by. My shaky 95-pound bench became as smooth and sure as an archer drawing a bow. "Strong!" said Dimitrios, grinning as he sidled past my bench while I finished a set. "You don't even need-a two finger!"

I even seemed to sweat less when I was carbed up with all that extra pasta and bread. I now understood how it felt to be the women I'd seen at that powerlifting meet all those years ago in Brooklyn, no longer a faint, glitchy hologram but instead solid and real, alive in all of my body from heart to fingertips.

One day, I decided I'd actually test the limits and eat as much food as I possibly could, just out of curiosity (at the time, it was trendy for influencers to attempt to eat 10,000 calories in a day and record it for YouTube or Instagram). On a Saturday morning, I ate my overnight oats and then planned out the day as an adventurous food tour through the Lower East Side: a huge fully loaded bagel with lox and cream cheese, two avocado toasts with chili oil and soy eggs, crackers and pimento cheese, a yeast donut stuffed with cornflake ice cream and drizzled with chocolate syrup. For good measure, I also had a protein shake. I ticked everything I ate into my calorie-tracking app as I lay, beached, on my couch. I hadn't even scratched 4,000 calories, and I felt like I was about to burst and splatter all over the walls of my apartment. I didn't know how the 10,000-calorie influencers were doing it, if they were faking it or using laxatives or what. But my body had limits, even if my imagination did not.

The biggest factor of all in bulking, though, was time. I could expect to gain, at best, only a few pounds of muscle in three months. It would take many years of hard training and eating a fairly specific diet—of trying as hard as I could to get big—just to gain even twenty pounds of muscle.

A lot of my confusion and fear about bulking stemmed from the inaccurate stories told in celebrity profiles promoting their upcoming movie. Actors "bulked up" for movie roles, and the headlines read that they gained 15, 20, 40 pounds of muscle in three months. Mickey Rourke claimed to gain 27 pounds of muscle in six months for *The Wrestler*. Emma Stone's trainer claimed she gained 15 pounds of muscle in three months for *Battle of the Sexes*. Gal Gadot claimed to gain 17 pounds of muscle in nine months for *Batman v Superman: Dawn of Justice*.

But these were all impossible tasks, especially without a lot of performance-enhancing drugs. Sure, it was possible to gain 27 or 15 or 17 pounds, period, in three or nine months. It was also possible for someone who had done a lot of dedicated strength training before to put muscle back on more quickly than it'd taken to build it the first time. But "20 pounds of muscle in three months" was just bad science communication by some poor sap who doesn't know a dumbbell from a barbell. By claiming these outsize effects, they made gaining muscle sound frighteningly easy. They also made it sound possible to gain a lot of muscle exclusively, yet another virtually impossible standard—building muscle requires a good-size margin of caloric error; otherwise, it doesn't take, and nothing happens. The framing also lightly implied that gaining muscle required a shift for the glamorous, famous person: *I wouldn't be caught dead gaining muscle* unless *it was to step outside myself and become someone else.*

Part of the reason the women that I'd found online were such a revelation is that many of them had tracked their bulks in real time. They might gain 15 or 20 pounds, but they were clear it was not all muscle, and that it shouldn't be. I was so used to before-and-after pictures being about weight loss, one body growing smaller after another. But in the before-and-afters of a bulk, everyone was visibly bigger—more muscular but, in their terms, "fluffier," too. Their weights had gone up, body weight *and* training weight, and they were delighted about it. They weren't doing it as a bit, or for some externalized purpose; they were doing it just because it was fun.

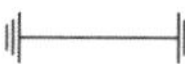

One day, I changed into my gym clothes, sliding off the jeans I'd had to jump in to get them up my legs and over my butt, and pulled on my leggings before heading to the gym. I was set to try and bench 110 pounds for one rep, three times, followed by four more upper-body accessory movements. On the second single rep, the barbell refused to fire off of my chest and instead dropped onto my sternum, lightly knocking the wind out of me. I sat there, not being crushed but not able to move, either. I mentally counted the days since my last period; I was, indeed, in the PMS window, which, despite my bulk, always sapped me of about 5 to 10 pounds' worth of strength. The gym was relatively quiet, and I'd failed so smoothly that no one seemed to even notice. No Dimitrios, no firefighters came to my aid. I wiggled the upper half of my body around, lightly panicking, before realizing I could just kind of lever my body and roll the barbell down my body until I could stand up. As I did so, I overhead two guys in the cable cross talking.

"Yeah, where's he at, man?"

"Some kind of heart issue," the other guy said, drying off the seat of the lat pull-down setup. "He's in the hospital." He paused. "Man, I wouldn't even be mad if his suitcase were here right now, man, no matter where he put it." I knew then they were talking about Dimitrios.

I felt a pang in my chest. My eyes welled up as I sat staring at my knees for a long time, transported back to the plain-white Best Buy bathroom where I'd been after I learned my dad had died. I knew Dimitrios was old. But his presence in the gym had been a near constant. He always seemed to arrive before me and left, presumably, after, though it was hard to know for sure because he was virtually always there, luggage and full-size cooler in tow as if he were making camp in the thicket of the gym.

I worried for him, being trapped somewhere with no weights, no coolers, interlocked with all the wrong kinds of machines. I knew barely anything about him, aside from his absolute dedication to barbell shrugs, his love for a good ringer tank. His unfailing kindness to me, no matter how unfriendly I was. I felt trapped by my lack of openness, my broken compass for other humans, my need to act out on other innocent people what I hadn't come to terms with, a need that interrupted the simple, pure, and good. I hoped Dimitrios was doing okay, surrounded by people who deserved him.

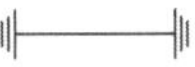

I came back to my apartment soaked in sweat after finishing the workout. My muscles pulsed with what Arnold Schwarzenegger once lasciviously described as "the pump," a tight, swelling feeling that seemed to come from them pressing on your skin from the inside. As I started making dinner, I caught sight of myself in the closet mirror. In the incomplete overhead light of my apartment, the shadows that fell on me seemed suddenly not just sharper, but larger. I'd grown. If I squeezed my upper arm and angled my forearm just right, I could see a bicep starting to form; if I pulled my arm across the front of my body just so, I could see just a hint of delt. My neck, which had previously perched above two sunken collarbones, now flowed into two triangular traps. I'd never felt more like an animal.

I had always internalized that being anything like an animal—raised by wolves, wild, uninhibited—was bad, unbecoming, unladylike. The right thing to do with those resemblances was to control them, straighten them out, push them down. The cultural disdain for being like an animal in any way was clear.

In my continuing research on the cultural history of strength, I wasn't surprised to learn that—while Christianity and lifting weights had dovetailed relatively recently in history—the war between Christianity and the animal body was ancient. Catholic theologian Thomas Aquinas's writings from the thirteenth century asserted that animal nature was contained in the essence of man, but only the parts of man that were *not* animal could be considered proof of God. That is, everything good and important about people, our immortal souls, was the basis for our religion and a divine gift, unlike our tawdry bodies. Not only that, denial of the body and its wants was in service of our souls, and of God. To give in to the body was to go against God. The attempt to separate us from our natural selves, to prevent us from inhabiting our bodies, to compartmentalize and isolate and operationalize our parts, was an old one. And now I saw why.

To be this big, to have and feel this much physical power, was a possibility I'd feared all my life. Except that where I'd always thought I'd see a monster, I saw a god, radiant like a big, beautiful horse. Doing everything I'd feared had allowed me to become exactly what I'd dreamed.

25

The Shirtdress

BACK WHEN MY JOB involved a lot of sprinting between PR events and reporting meetings, I had a go-to outfit that walked the line of reasonably put-together and professional but plausibly workaday: a pair of stretchy, skinny black pants with jeans-style pockets, and a chambray shirt. I wore that trusty chambray shirt all over, from LA to Vegas to launches for chintzy Android phones in Hell's Kitchen. It was the perfect uniform. But the first time I put the shirt on after starting to bulk, it felt tight, particularly in the arms. I turned away from the mirror and absentmindedly reached one elbow up behind my head to scratch between my shoulder blades, when I heard a rip. I turned back to the mirror. The sleeve had torn on the underside of my upper arm, from armpit to elbow. I had accidentally Hulked out of my shirt.

I'd recently bought a brand-new pair of skinny black Madewell jeans and paid precious dollars to get them tailored to bring in the waist, so that they'd fit me like a glove. But after a few months of wearing them, the already-too-thin and soft denim fabric had started to wear out between my legs. One day, I brought a knee up too high above my waist, and the pants ripped knee to crotch, the two halves flapping open to reveal half my thigh.

The process of my muscles getting bigger was not so different from when I'd been doing recomposition: I was training to shred my muscle fibers and then eating enough food and protein to repair them to the degree that they were slightly better and ever so slightly bigger than before. In a few weeks, I wouldn't have gained more than a couple pounds of muscle, which would look like two eight-ounce steak filets side by side.

It is not known exactly why muscles work this way—why they are able to be damaged, why the response is to repair them in such a way that they're even better than they were before, increasing the number of myofibrils within each muscle fiber. But muscle protein synthesis, the process that builds muscle, is dictated by our genetic code and requires the cooperation of many moving parts. How well we synthesize protein into muscle is dependent not just on the amount of available protein, but also on carbohydrates, nutrients, timing, hydration, and more. Still, with all of the available material, it happens automatically. Our best biological theory is that our bodies repair muscles this way, better than before, in an effort to protect them from further damage. If it hurt us this time, we'll build the walls twice as high and thick so it won't happen again.

But even as my body was getting more resilient, I wished my muscles didn't need to sacrifice my clothes to prove it. These kinds of incidents were not constant, but they were enough to form a trend. One clothing loss, though, really stuck out.

It is a truth of shopping at H&M that when you find a piece of clothing where there's only one size left and it's your size, you are ordained to buy it, because clearly everyone else did already, and that's market wisdom you can trust. On one trip to H&M long ago, I'd found a beautiful, crisp, pin-striped long-sleeved shirtdress, the kind of thing one might wear to attend the US Open. Instead of falling straight like a true shirtdress, it had a skirt with many pleats, slightly shorter on the sides than in the front and back. I was snatched for the gods in this dress; well, except in the chest, where my boobs wrenched the button placket apart a little. I resolved to pin the placket in place and bought the dress.

One day in 2014, right around the time I started to lift but before my body had started to evolve, I was wearing the dress on a date in the dusky heat of the rising New York summer. As we lingered outside the IFC theater in the West Village, I saw a familiar face emerge: a glamorous D-list celebrity I recognized from the *Bachelor* universe, on the arm of an equally handsome man. She noticed me staring and stared back at me as her path intersected with ours. "Are you—?" I said.

"Yes." She smiled and then looked me excitedly up and down. "*Where* did you get your dress?"

"H&M," I said in my best this-old-thing voice.

"I love it," she said, and twirled away with her date. From then on, I wore it as often as a pin-striped, pleated seersucker shirtdress made sense.

But as I continued to lift weights, my body started straining all of the buttons until they gapped; the armpits pinched; my butt lifted the skirt just enough that it became dangerously short for a city prone to random gusts of wind. I stopped wearing the dress, but for years, I kept it in my closet as a trophy.

One day, I was looking for a picture of myself in the dress, and I scrolled back to the end of 2013. I landed on a picture I'd taken from before I'd started lifting, standing in a Lululemon dressing room stall while I'd been trying on some clothes. I was transported into the memory of taking that photo, how I'd been trying to hold my arms and torso in the mirror so they appeared as thin as possible. I'd been happy with the photo then, a rare occurrence. But looking at it now, three years later, I saw a different person.

I looked emaciated, delicate, like I could snap, an oversize head with sunken cheeks and eyes and big hands swimming atop a vanishing body. What I'd looked at and been pleased to see years ago horrified me now. I'd always believed I'd never had any real results from dieting or working out, insisted that I couldn't possibly be unhealthy because nothing had *really* worked as well as it was supposed to. Here, I was confronted with evidence that not only had I been wrong, but I hadn't been able to *see* how wrong I was. I scrolled back through more photos of myself that I knew I'd reflexively hated, but the time and events that had gone by had dissolved the perceived distortions. She had been a beautiful girl, but had also already been everything my warped brain had wanted so desperately. It was even more stark how everything inside and outside of me had worked to rob me of every ounce of connection to reality.

I had already, spiritually, kissed goodbye my desire to be skinny when I started bulking, but I hadn't completely let go. That day, I added the dress to my pile of donation clothes, leaving the clip I'd sewn in to close the boob gap. Then I bought a new dress, a saloon-goes-boho one in a dark-green floral pattern, cut high in the front and low in the back, with a ruffled hem and cap sleeves that could slide off my shoulders and expose the full span of my upper back. One day, I wore it to the *New York Times* office and met my friend Mike for lunch. As we got up and he followed me to put up our trays, I heard "Whoa—your back is *huge*!" I smiled. I knew "huge" was relative; Schwarzenegger was huge. But I hadn't thought about my back in a while. That night, I turned in circles after getting out of the shower, trying to crane my neck to see behind me in the reflection. There were new shadows that hadn't always been there, that serpentined and intertwined from the tops of my shoulders down to the small of my back. In the old long-sleeved shirtdress, they would have been concealed. The new dress put them under the light. It struck me then that the expression for being confident and brave was "having some backbone," when in fact, the bones, plural, of my back did very little. If I finally had some backbone, it had nothing to do with the bones; it was the muscles.

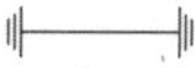

After three months, I could feel my strength gains slowing down again, but I loved bulking so much, the feeling of having wings in the gym, that I didn't want to stop. So I decided to push it for an additional month. I raised my calories again, from 2,760 to 3,150, and finally from 3,150 to 3,500 calories every day. Even with the increased calories, my weight gain slowed down. I eked out a little more lifting progress, edging in some additional reps and adding a few more pounds to my lifts here and there. But as the fourth month came to a close, I was surprised to find I was getting tired of all the eating; the logistics of never missing a meal; trying to beat my appetite to the punch and finish all my food before the fullness set in; and just all of the chewing, constant, endless chewing. I longed for a simple meal I could eat at my ponderous pace, stop when I was full, and think no more about. I didn't want to anticipate and plan for the next snack in a couple of hours, and yet another sizable meal beyond that.

I'd never in my life expected eating a lot to become in any way unfun; I thought there was no limit to how much I could enjoy food, in quantity or otherwise. I'd really, really never expected it to become a chore from which I longed to be excused. At the same time, the hold that food had had over me was now long gone. A brownie was a brownie; a cube of cheese was a cube of cheese.

From that moment, the bulking experiment was over. I weighed 165 pounds, about 12 pounds more than when I started. By that time, all of my lifting numbers had gone up dramatically: I could squat 220 pounds for one rep, which brought me tantalizingly close to the "two plates" benchmark of 225. I'd switched to a different style of deadlifting—sumo—that felt like it didn't demand as much of my lower back, and despite having to learn another style, I'd posted three singles at 240 pounds. I could bench 120 pounds, which put me within spitting distance of benching the "full plate" of 135 pounds.

I was as heavy as I'd ever been, even a few pounds heavier than the highest weight I'd reached in college that had precipitated my yearslong downward spiral into cardio and dieting. As I'd filled out with muscle, my proportions changed: I had bigger legs and arms, a bigger back, and to my surprise, more "abs" than I'd ever seen when I weighed far less and did only core workouts. But more than that, the harmonious feedback loop of eating and training was radiating into my feelings about myself. Taking care of myself helped me see that I was worth taking care of. I had limits, and they weren't something to be ashamed of; knowing the limits was what made everything else work.

I'd always known something about my physical existence wasn't working, and I'd been determined to attack my body until I tortured the answer out of it. I was my own most acutely attuned hater under the guise of being my most dedicated protector from criticism. When I started lifting, before starting to bulk, I'd also tried like hell to release any expectation of liking how I looked at all, hoping that with enough detachment, I could speed through it and get back to losing body fat again. But after committing the sinful act of weight gain and strength building and bulking, I loved what I saw in the mirror. My appearance's conformity and how I felt about it, I saw now, were two concepts that had nothing to do with each other. How I felt about myself had nothing to do with my weight, or my shape, or even how much fat or muscle I had; it was whether I allowed my body to be the home it should be and always was.

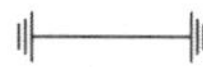

I hadn't developed any real close relationships at Richie's; mostly it was nodding acknowledgment and the briefest of chats when equipment changed hands. For the most part, we were all each focused on what was going on in our headphones, and that suited me fine. But one day, as I was exiting the gym and sorting out a membership renewal at the front desk, a regular member passed by as he was entering. He was wearing a muscle tank and was about my height, but he was one of the larger and leaner bros, with thinning hair and a face whose veins and crags betrayed years and years of straining for those last few reps to failure. "You come here a lot, right?" he said, catching my eye.

"Yes! For a couple years now," I said.

"I've been watching you," he said, smiling. "You look good. You look *strong*."

"Wow, thank you!" I said. I looked at the front-desk guy, who smiled in the same way. The gymgoer high-fived me and said, "Keep it up!" before ambling away.

Finally, I thought with a hint of irony, *someone noticed*. But more feelings sloshed around inside me; I'd always struggled with the feeling of being unkindly watched, like there was someone always waiting for me to fuck up and put me in my place, someone waiting with a "Nice job! But..." or worse, a "I can't believe you just..." There had been a couple such interlopers.

And yet here had been this guy, and maybe many more in the gym—Dimitrios, the firefighters, people who'd watched me try and fail over and over, who'd seen me wind my way from fumbling around with 10-pound dumbbells to loading up 240 pounds on my deadlift. They'd trusted that my hapless little journey of trying to do anything at all in the gym would unfold as it needed to, that I'd keep showing up and the weights would do what weights did. It was a kind of trust I'd never felt before, that I could handle it, but also that there was no need to indoctrinate me or tell me what to think; what would need to happen would happen.

As I walked out the swinging glass door, I thought about the last few years. After spending so long fighting for some basic amount of peace, my drive toward discomfort had turned out to be a double-edged sword. It was as if, before lifting, I had been in quicksand thrashing around, abandoning myself in a futile effort not to drown. It wasn't until I slowed down and stayed in myself, making slower and more deliberate movements, that I started to work my way out.

Maybe I might never really change—I might always be wary, distrustful, trapped in my own head to some degree. The foundations of my relationship to the world had been wired into my very neurons before I was even fully conscious. Anywhere I went, anything I did, I could only begin from myself. I was the person I needed to hold my own hands and see and feel and know all the ways I could be and know what I needed. I wasn't sure I deserved the credit for changing, exactly. What had really happened was that I'd become something more like myself.

26

Generations

IT WAS THE THANKSGIVING after my first bulk, and high off my newly gained muscle, I was trying to do the impossible: talk my mother into trying to lift weights. In an appeal to her eternal concern about how much she weighed, I tried to defy her expectations of what weight looked like.

"You look like you've gained some weight," she said in a tone I imagine she thought sounded neutral.

"Guess how much I weigh," I said to her.

"A hundred and sixty-five pounds," she guessed, perfectly accurately.

She'd always been a staunch exerciser, jogging with two or four of us kids piled into a bicycle-wheeled stroller and then tracking the length of the jog by retracing it with the odometer in the car. Though she'd never been more than a size six, she'd also always been a dedicated dieter, grapefruits in the morning and only an appetizer (spinach-and-artichoke dip) when we went out for dinner. But she also loved food: everything bagels with a layer of butter and then peanut butter, Breyers ice cream with Hershey's syrup that she'd binge until she was overwhelmed with guilt. She even performed restriction with her car, putting gas in only five dollars at a time when our budget was thinnest, the tank always hovering near empty.

My mother regarded my lifting with a wary curiosity that stopped short of interest. She'd been lifting weights all her life in the form of her constantly growing children—we'd cling to her shins as she tried to walk around, sit on her like a horse while she tried to buck us off, and she'd pick us up and carry us out of a store if need be—but she didn't see this in herself. The closest thing to conventional weights in our house growing up had been some canvas Velcro ankle weights that must have come with a Jane Fonda DVD.

But I felt sure I could convert her. Lifting was essential for older women, preserving their lean mass and strengthening their bones. But aside from the straightforward benefits, I hoped it would instigate the realization that she didn't actually want what she thought she did, that perhaps dieting was making her into an even more rigid, stressed-out, unhappy person than she was aware of. She had been baiting me into managing her feelings her whole life, but at long last I felt like I might actually be up to the job.

I went with her to the gym where she was a member to teach her some basics. We ran through one day's worth of movements—squat, bench, rows. The whole time she was glancing nervously at me, like one might at a jailer. "That's good," I said during her squats. "Try not to arch your back so much; you just want it to be straight."

"It bothers my knees," she said, doing another rep.

"Well, the way you have your knees would kind of strain them. Try it more like this."

"But my knees aren't supposed to go past my toes."

"They can! That's a myth."

"Says who?"

"Says, I don't know, everything I've ever read."

"Well, everything *I've* ever read says the opposite."

"Well, your knees hurt when you do it your way. Don't you think that means it might not work?"

"Maybe it just doesn't work for me because there's something wrong with my knees."

"Mom, there's nothing wrong with your knees."

"You don't know that; you're not a doctor."

It went on like this until we reached the end.

"And that's it?" she said.

"That's it!"

"But I'm not even sweating."

"That's okay; you don't have to sweat in order to get a good workout."

"But I always sweat when I've had a good workout."

"Well, lifting is different."

"Okay. I'm just—" She glanced in the direction of the floor mats across from a couple of leg-raise stands. "I'm just going to go do my core." Before I could say anything, she turned and went to one of the mats and proceeded to do thirty minutes of crunches, planks, leg raises, and a number of other moves I didn't even recognize. I sighed and went back to my bench.

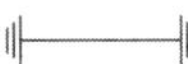

When we got home, I typed her numbers into a total-daily-energy-expenditure calculator—using height, weight, age, activity level—and showed her the results. "See? This is how much you should be eating every day," I said.

She looked at the screen, then warily back at me, and smiled tightly. "But I feel full on twelve hundred calories," she said. "If I eat more than that, I gain weight."

"But you don't really!" I said and tried to explain the way that people can retain water with new amounts of food or new workouts, that it can settle out after several days, the way that having dieted too much for too long lowers people's metabolisms. "You might be able to eat way more than you are, and nothing would even change!"

She smiled tightly some more. "Okay," she said hesitantly now, as if I had broken into her house and brandished a knife at her. "I don't see how that could be, when I gain weight when I eat. When I eat too much, I gain three pounds the next day."

I put my head in my hands. There was no way she of the 1,200 daily calories was accidentally eating an additional 11,000 calories' worth of food to make her actually gain three pounds in a day. These were the same misunderstandings I'd had. I would have killed to have someone pierce the veil and help me live a different way. Why wouldn't she let me? Why did she have no interest, no belief, no trust in anything I was saying?

The truth was, as I thought about it, I was up against old, deeply worn beliefs. As an adult, I had learned more about how she might have developed this kind of mindset. My grandmother, her mother, had been the subject of their small town's morbid fascination, essentially the town crazy. They nicknamed her Wacky Jackie, and she was someone you did not meet or know as much as survive. She subsisted on coffee and suspicion and penny-pinched her way up and down Main Street. She made all her daughters' clothes as if it were still the Great Depression and viciously warned them to stay away from their home's windows. No one would ever know exactly what bedeviled Wacky Jackie; she died when I was six years old. But the fact that my own mother didn't live as a recluse, avoiding the windows of her own home, was a testament to her own internal fight. I found out that she, too, had become a runner in college, a practice she continued to the present day.

Still, I felt like my contentment and ease about food and working out was shining through my skin. Eating more and working out differently had lifted my anxiety and eased the desperation and trepidation I felt about physically existing in the world. I was the happiest I'd ever been. But I knew, at root, that my mom didn't trust my ability to know what happiness was, that she thought I was operating under a kind of delusion. She had her own mother's suspicion. It was as if I were telling her I weighed less because I now lived on the moon, or that I owed my health to little green men who tractor-beamed me into their spaceship each night.

It hurt that she didn't trust me, not only as a living, breathing example of all the things I was saying, but as her daughter who cared about her, who wanted her to live a long time, and who—most importantly—wanted more than anything to see her be kind to herself, for the first time ever.

I had watched her struggle mightily for a modicum of peace and happiness all my life. But even when she got on the right track, she seemed compelled to undercut herself. I was desperate for her to relent, to release the rules she held so tightly, that were so hostile to her. The facts of how things could be better felt so simple and near to the surface. But what felt simple and near to the surface for me, I suppose, felt to her like it was in deep, unexplored space.

"What is it you're afraid of?" I asked. "Even if you tried this and it turned out you did gain three pounds, why would that be so bad?"

She paused, then smiled apologetically, painfully. "I don't want to be one of those fat old women," she said.

"But even if that's what three pounds did, which it wouldn't," I said, "why would that be so bad?"

"No one likes fat old women."

"I can think of lots of fat old women that many people love."

"But they wouldn't love me."

I looked at her. I wanted to tell her, *Yes, they would*. But of all the things I was saying and she wasn't believing, it would be the one she would believe the least. She was working so hard to deserve love but couldn't bring herself to open the door. She had scarcely dated since divorcing my dad almost twenty years before, and she mostly kept to herself. When she made new connections, they never seemed to be able to measure up to her standards. I could argue my case until I turned blue, and it wouldn't change the fundamental unlovableness that she believed about herself, or that unlovableness was the consequence of gaining three whole pounds.

I sighed. "I wish I could make you know that that's not true."

"Well, I'm just stupid, I guess."

"Jesus," I said, standing up. I'd tried. "I love you. If you change your mind, you know how to reach me."

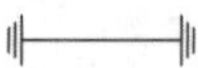

One day I finally corralled my friend Emma into Richie's to learn to bench. "You don't need your feet so far apart," I said. "That's better. Grab the bar out here; your hands are a little close. Now push it up and out." She strained, and nothing happened. "Here—" I went to go around the other side to help her, when all of a sudden, Dimitrios appeared behind the rack. It was the first time I'd seen him since I'd heard about his heart issue. I'd been worried, but I didn't want to intrude on his business. I was relieved to see he betrayed zero signs of unwellness at all; he was his usual, genial, gregarious self. "She a-show you!" he said, yelling over the music at Emma, pointing to me and then to her. Emma sat up and turned in his direction, then jumped a little when she saw him.

"She show you!" Dimitrios said, pointing again. "Strong!" he said, pointing at me and making a muscle.

"Okay," she said sarcastically, turning back to me as Dimitrios lumbered past, grinning to himself.

"No—it's okay," I said, smiling. "He's fine. He's just here a lot. We see each other a lot. He means well." I turned to ask him a million questions, both because I was curious and concerned about what had happened to him and because I was hoping to make up for Emma's attitude. But he was already on the other side of the room, his back to us with headphones on and busying himself with his shrugs. I watched him for a moment. The weight he was lifting even seemed the same as it had always been, a nearly uncountable number of plates on each side. If he'd had a heart issue, it had been no match for his body, or maybe just his attitude.

He shrugged the barbell ten times, then slammed it back onto the safety arms with a huge BANG that rattled through the big room. Emma winced, bringing her hands to her ears. "Geeeez," she said under her breath. "Take it easy."

I laughed. "Well, remember when you said you were afraid to even clink the plates because you felt like you were being too loud?"

"Yeah," Emma said.

"Now you see," I said, "if you make some noise, you're not alone. Everyone's banging things."

"I'll never make as much noise as that guy."

"Come on—don't be so hard on yourself," I said, shaking her shoulder, before grasping it as if searching for muscle. "How many calories are you eating now?"

"Twenty-five hundred."

"Don't lie to me."

"Okay—eighteen hundred calories."

"Em-ma."

"I can't eat any more! I get so full!"

"What are you eating? What did you eat yesterday?"

"Granola...farro..." She was trailing off. "Salad..."

"After this, we are going to eat burgers."

"I can't!"

"Burger or no bench!"

"Hey, I thought you can't use food as a carrot."

"Well, now the food is the stick. Now let's lie down again."

"You can't make me eat the burger."

"I can't make you do anything—you are a big girl. If you want to do all these beautiful bench reps and then piss them away on some salad greens, that is your business."

She smirked. "I'm going to earn my burger," she said, knowing it would annoy me.

"No being toxic while benching," I said, pointing to the rack. She lay down and grabbed the barbell again.

27

The Worst-Ever Date Ever

IN 2018, FOUR YEARS after I'd started lifting, I was on a first date I was not enjoying at all. We were at a bar near my apartment, when the guy rested his hand on my leg. It wasn't on the knee but higher up and on the side of my thigh, almost on my hip. I was so bewildered I didn't react, and he left his hand sitting there for many seconds, until he had to remove it to gesture.

"Of course, the Saint A's parties were second to none," he explained to me, waving his hands around. Saint A's was a chichi fraternity-like club at Columbia, where we'd both gone to college. Why he felt like he had to explain Saint A's, an organization as notorious for its free-flowing cocaine as its parties, I had no idea. Everyone I knew at Columbia knew what Saint A's was, but none had ever expended a single breath in its direction, let alone done free PR for its supposedly legendary parties.

I studied his face as he continued selling me on the private club of the school I also went to. "What year did you graduate again?" I said. He had claimed to be twenty-eight in his dating profile.

"Ah...two thousand," he said, grimacing a little. This man was fully ten years older than his app profile had said. But he blustered on. "So what is this place? It's corny," he said, motioning around.

"It's a tiki bar. They have a lot of different kinds of rum," I said.

"Who drinks rum?" he said. "You know, you only need one rum. Do you know which rum that is?"

"No," I said.

"Captain Morgan. Captain Morgan is the best rum; everything else is—" He waved his arm in a dismissive gesture at all the bottles behind the bar. The bartender, attracted or alarmed by the man who kept swinging his arms, came over. "Can I get a Captain Morgan? Do you even *have* Captain Morgan? Captain Morgan on the rocks, and that's it," he said.

"Rum old-fashioned," I said.

"Ooooh," he said to me, wiggling his fingers in an aren't-you-fancy gesture.

The bartender made up the drinks. My date took a big gulp of his Captain Morgan. "Ahhh," he said theatrically. "You just can't beat it!"

I sipped my drink, trying to take as big a swig as I could without swallowing all of the ice, hoping for a little relief. If you have the specific goal of trying to find a compatible partner and committing to one another, dating in New York is hell on Earth. I did want a boyfriend, though, and the anonymous nature of app-based dating gave me the courage I'd never had. Maybe too much. There seemed to be so many strange and exotic humans who had washed onto the shores of the city, often in a bubble of their own ignorance made of their parents' money.

Viewed not as a mission but instead as a safari, dating was some of the most fun I could have. I could see the jerks more clearly now and even was fascinated by them. Sometimes I stuck around longer than I needed to, just out of journalistic curiosity. I liked to think I could put on a charming enough front to make this work, most of the time.

I drained my drink until the ice was dry. "I have to go to the bathroom," I said, and escaped off the stool. When I sat back down not two minutes later, I looked at the glass and shook the ice around. The ice of my previously empty drink didn't click but slosh; it appeared suspiciously wet. I looked from the drink to him; he was scrolling on his phone, face buried in his second Captain Morgan. Ice didn't melt that fast. Was this motherfucker trying to roofie me?

I pushed the glass away to the bartender's side. My date looked up. "You're back," he said. "So what about these rums?" He paused before gesturing again to the bar's shelves. "What here do you think is better than Captain Morgan?" Before I could answer, he turned to the bartender.

"What's the best rum in your opinion?" he said, talking to the bartender, "of all the ones you have?"

"Flor de Caña," the bartender said, betraying no emotion. Flor de Caña was thirty-two dollars a pour.

"Let's have it," he said. The bartender obligingly poured another shot in a ceramic glass shaped like an upside-down pineapple. My date sipped it. "It all tastes the same!" he exclaimed. "Here—try it."

"I'm good," I said.

"Aghhh," he said, waving his hands in dissatisfaction. As he got progressively drunker, I realized that in another time, I would have felt responsible for, even guilty over, this display, given that I was the one he was trying to prove a point to. Now I could enjoy the moment for what it really was: some guy making an ass of himself. Eventually I said it was time to go, and with a wan, resigned look, he slid off his chair and followed me outside.

"So what now?" he said.

"Thank you for the drinks," I said.

"Want to go to the Upper East Side? I know a great bar near my place," he said. I hadn't told him how close my own place was—a secret I intended to keep forever.

"I have to go," I said, "but it was great to meet you." I turned to go, but he grabbed my elbow, gently at first. I reflexively tugged to pull it away, and although he was many drinks deeper than I was, his reflex was just as fast—instead of letting me go, his hand tightened.

Before I could even think, I swung my left hand up toward his cheek. I intended to slap him across the face, but my whole body ratcheted into motion as if I were throwing a pitch at Yankee Stadium, winding up my hip and through my upper body and whipping them through their rotation. My hand connected with such force and frantic aim that I ended up clubbing him upside the head with my hand and most of my forearm. He spun halfway around and folded toward the ground, emitting a long, rising wail. "Sorry!" I said, flabbergasted, and before he could recover, I turned and ran, dashing around the corner toward my apartment. I checked behind me, and he wasn't following. I didn't stop running until I reached my door. I'd never been so happy to not know my own strength.

28

Cutting

THE LAST FEW YEARS of lifting had gone better than I'd ever dreamed. The muscle I hadn't even known I'd lost with all that dieting now blanketed my bones like armor. My own sense of strength still hadn't caught up to reality, so I'd prepare to put effort into picking up a big bag or box before walking over to it and lifting it in the air like Michael Jordan palming a basketball. Because of that, I was in a near-constant state of surprise and delight.

Contrary to my wild fears, things had not spun out of control while I'd been bulking. I was happily carrying around a bunch of body fat while building up more muscle. But the effects of bulking had worn off after a few months: my strength progress had slowed down, and I no longer felt the glorious energy during my gym sessions that I once did, and I was tired of eating. Now if I wanted to be able to bulk again, I'd have to lose the body fat I'd gained to reset the bulking clock.

Weight loss had always gone hand in hand with resenting my body, wanting to destroy it for its shortcomings and inconveniences—and then gaining weight had gone from my nightmare to my saving grace. What would happen if I tried to make there be less of me again? I'd managed to wrangle the related demons into a closet and lock it. Going near the door again seemed like a bad idea.

I had gained, I guessed, probably eight to ten pounds of body fat over the course of my bulk. "Cutting" was the counterpart to "bulking," where I would shed the body fat I gained while doing everything I could to hold on to the new muscle I had built. Losing this body fat would restore my appetite and put me back in a position to bulk, build even more muscle and strength, and do the whole cycle all over again. That was the real goal. As I knew from disastrous experience, it was possible to lose muscle, a lot of it, by indiscriminately eating too little, which could set off a chain reaction of negative consequences. I wasn't at immediate risk of that anymore, but I did want to keep the results of my hard work.

"Cutting" and "bulking" are not common terminology, but they are familiar terms to any athlete trying to put on muscle. Usually, these cuts and bulks are interrupted by periodic cycles of "maintenance" to help the results of the last cycle stick. Over the course of a few years, athletes can put on dozens of pounds of muscle by cycling between these phases; without performance-enhancing drugs, it's the fastest process for building muscle that exists.

To not lose weight so fast that I'd lose muscle, too, I had to keep eating a lot of protein: a gram per pound of body weight—for me, 165 grams a day. But I also had to be careful not to eat too little. In fact, I was trying to *eat as much as possible,* while still steadily losing the body fat I'd gained. My books cautioned that a calorie deficit greater than 25 percent or so would put my muscle at risk and cause unnecessary suffering. This meant I couldn't lose more than a pound or so per week.

Hoping to avoid suffering entirely, I started with a 15 percent deficit to be safe. My maintenance calories were around 2,400, so this meant to start losing body fat, I'd go down to 2,040 calories. I hoped it worked; Oprah would faint dead away at the idea of someone trying to lose weight on this many calories. I also hoped things wouldn't get out of control, knowing now that equilibrium was possible, and equilibrium included some body fat.

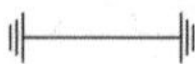

Bodies have an awareness of how much fat they have, because fat plays crucial roles, and those roles are not, as many diet explainers only grudgingly admit, just insulation and energy storage. Body fat stores vitamins (A, D, E, and K); coats nerves and connective tissues; and regulates hormones, including estrogen, insulin, and cortisol. Certain immune cells found in fat are even anti-inflammatory. While body fat is more flexible in quantity than most other kinds of tissue in the body—that is, we can store it and burn it more easily than, say, bone or organ mass—its presence is still critical for all of those essential bodily functions. This is one reason why bodies work so hard to manipulate energy levels and metabolism to prevent from losing too much body fat too quickly and, in a lot of cases, seem to work uphill against any kind of change in body-composition status quo: complex systems threaten to shut down when bodies don't have all the fat they need.

To understand what happens at the extremes of body-fat manipulation, it can help to look at body builders. No one is better at manipulating body fat than a body builder, and they have the skills to push body-fat loss to the absolute limit. When body builders get on stage, their goal is always to be as lean as possible, with their skin virtually shrink-wrapped to their muscles. In order to accomplish this, they use extremely meager diets, sometimes subsisting on only a few hundred meticulously counted calories per day, in the days leading up to the show (this is referred to as "peaking"). In almost every case, it's impossible for women to get down to less than 10 percent body fat and sustain it without suffering immediate and extreme consequences: loss of their period, severe mood swings, sleep disruption, sexual dysfunction, and exhaustion. Long term, low body fat and the resulting affected biology and hormones cause osteoporosis. Even less than 15 percent body fat can begin to produce some of these effects.

Around the time I started lifting, a number of the women I could find online who lifted were body builders, many of them specifically competing in a new division called "bikini" that had been created for women with less-muscular figures. One of the most popular body-builder influencers, Nikki Blackketter, would post videos of herself preparing for various bikini shows, including the smaller and smaller meals she would eat leading up to show day in order to make her muscles and veins bulge through her thinned skin. In one of her "peak week" videos from 2015, she showed herself eating a meal that included only a small plate of chicken, a cup of berries, and a low-fat yogurt. In a video from the day before the competition, she showed herself eating only a rice cake, stating that she was tempted to put a little ketchup on it because she was so desperate to eat something with any flavor. "I'm super ready...I'm ready to eat again, and not be hungry anymore," she told the camera wanly the night before her show.

But as distantly as she spoke of her continued diet, she spoke reverently, excitedly, in anticipation of eating once the competition was over, even to the point of scarfing junk food. Though her goal was to be extremely lean on stage, it was never her intent to stay that way for longer than a matter of hours; being so lean was way too miserable.

Men are able to access slightly lower levels of body fat due to a different distribution—5 percent tends to be their lower limit—but they suffer the same effects. As the body-fat-manipulation protocols of body builders have spread over the internet, more and more bros try them out, working hard in the gym to be attractive to "chicks," exercising and dieting and getting so shredded that their veins pop out of their skin. But the leanness they achieve turns out to be a gift of the magi: once they are so shredded, their hormones are so out of whack that they lose all interest in having sex and even can't maintain an erection, due to how depleted their bodies are. It's been rare for the professional hot people of the world to speak candidly about this, though some have begun to. Of his process of losing body fat for *Magic Mike's Last Dance*, Channing Tatum said, "It's not natural.... You have to starve yourself. I don't think when you're that lean it's actually healthy for you." Comedian Eric André lost forty-five pounds for the sixth season of his TV show and told *Men's Health*, "If you see any middle-aged person with abs know that they're either psychotic or unemployed, because it is a full time job."

I'd heard all about the negative effects that can be correlated with higher body fat: heart disease, diabetes, cancer. In extreme cases, higher body fat—in the category defined as class III obesity—is correlated with an upward trend in overall mortality. But body fat itself is not a complete measure of health in either direction. Often, it is presented as a lockstep metric—the less body fat, the more health, and vice versa. As research and medicine have started to use a more weight-inclusive approach in studying health and longevity, scientists have uncovered that "more than the bare amount of necessary body fat" is far from some kind of glaring red emergency beacon. The dangers of body fat in and of itself are vastly oversold; meanwhile, how essential body fat is to functioning simply never gets discussed.

I had tried to chase down my own body fat like a villager with a pitchfork, only to find that arranging my life that way left me both mentally and physically miserable. In the world of strength training, it was not obligatory to either lose all of one's body fat or keep it all. What mattered most was that if someone did want to lose body fat, the process deserved some respect and care, so that it didn't harm their livelihood, their muscles, or their sanity.

29

The Deceptively Elusive Pull-Up

NOW THAT I WAS cutting, I woke up some mornings, rolled out of bed, and pulled my bathroom scale out into the kitchen / living room / office where there was actually room to use it. I weighed myself every few days and logged it in a spreadsheet. Thanks to hormones and fluids, the graph was all peaks and valleys, but with a little spreadsheet magic, a downward trend line emerged. As I gradually lost body fat, muscle definition emerged that I'd never seen before: calves, elbows, abs. The seedlings of my muscles, fertilized by the extra calories and body fat of my bulk, had turned to fruit.

Getting all of my protein did become a little more difficult with fewer calories to spread it around in. I ate leaner meats, like chicken breasts or fish instead of hamburgers or pork shoulder. Exchanging whole-fat yogurt and milk for low or nonfat gave me a hundred extra calories to play around with. Overall, the changes were minimal, and the meals just slightly smaller; my plates had a little less rice and fewer potatoes and a little more meat. Embarrassing though it was, I kept sugar-free Jell-O in the fridge and rice cakes around to eat if I felt like chewing on something.

I found that eating enough fat could be the difference between feeling really hungry and not feeling any particular cravings. But I also discovered the hard way that, with limited carbs, I'd pay for every rep. A couple of weeks in, without the extra calories of bulking to carry me through, I started pouring sweat during my workouts, soaking through my shirts and shorts. Any time I lay down or sat on a bench, I left an anatomically graphic sweat print.

"You work hard, yes?" said Dimitrios, grinning while I was keeled over between sets of rows, sweat rolling from within my scalp down my forehead and into my eyebrows. I had tried eating fifty fewer grams of carbs that day.

"Uh-huh" was all I could manage, though I smiled to him.

"You extend," said Dimitrios, showing me his own arm rowing but letting his shoulder round forward toward the ground before retracting the whole joint and pulling back up.

"Uh-huh," I said, nodding. "Okay."

"You work hard," said Dimitrios again, smiling. "Very good. Very, very good." He ambled away.

I knew enough to expect progress at the gym to stall while I was eating less, and that the best I could hope for was to maintain where I was at. When I got my period about a month into my cut, my weight spiked up four pounds for several days. The few pounds of body-fat loss, designed to be so slow and gradual, had appeared to be completely erased by random events. I gritted my teeth at the spreadsheet but resolved not to do anything. A few days later, the graph dipped down again by 5.5 pounds.

I had never lost weight by any method other than severe deprivation and raw determination, skipping as many meals as I could and eating as little as possible when I did have to eat. The idea was that, even if the process was brutal, the harder I could be on myself, the sooner it would be over. I used to weigh myself night and day, horrified every night when I appeared to have gained several pounds throughout the day even when I'd worked extremely hard to barely eat. Now I'd come to understand that as the least significant fluctuation of all: bodies rehydrate and refuel with food through the day, then get dehydrated and depleted overnight while we aren't eating. Dietary ghosts. To smooth out the data, I only weighed myself "dry" in the mornings.

Through all this, the old compulsions I feared might be triggered by dieting, by tracking, by weighing—in hopes of weight loss—did not show up. Eating less did not make me feel compelled to eat even less still; knowing that it would hurt to try and hurry the process, and that the process was working exactly as quickly as it should—which was actually pretty slowly—kept me on the path. Again, I found that it was possible to do what I wanted in a much easier way, without starving, without agony over fluctuations. I'd been taught not to trust my body with any resources at all, that its system was primed to betray me, that to manage it and take care of it was to fight it, hard. I'd treated myself like a big, dumb beast of burden.

Now, years later, I had arrived back at my own beginning, with that old goal of trying to lose weight. But every conceivable thing about it was different. It wasn't painful. It wasn't about fighting myself. It was taking advantage of how my body already worked, its desire to preserve muscle, its ability to use body fat as fuel in small increments. Most important of all, the goal was no longer even to be skinny; it was to restore my sensitivity to calories, to reorient so that I could get back to bulking, eating, and my glorious carb-fueled gym sessions again that made me stronger. I didn't even remotely plan to stay lean. As soon as I reached the bottom of the valley, I was impatient to turn right around and hike back up the hill again.

Toward the end of the cut, my energy had finally been strained a little by all the weeks of moderated food, and my lifting numbers had started to wobble. I hated any backward movement, still. But the concept of "muscle memory" I'd always heard about, it turned out, didn't just apply to things like riding a bike. It also applied to lifting. Now that I'd gone through all of these months, and now years, of training, my nervous system had had these movement patterns carved into them, and my muscles had built up. If I were to suddenly stop, it would all slowly fade away—the strength, the physical muscles. But if after a long break, I started lifting again, everything would come back again much faster than it had taken to learn the first time, because that imprint never truly leaves. Research shows that the very cells of skeletal muscle appear to develop a "memory" of strength, of the contractions performed during lifting. The effects of lifting are epigenetic: even if I stopped lifting, it was now written into my DNA. Even if I didn't stay as strong as I was then forever, the strength I had built was always going to be there, going to be a part of me, going to be mine.

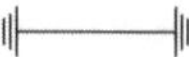

There was one goal that had eluded me all this time. A few years before, I'd read with great interest an article in the *New York Times* headlined "Why Women Can't Do Pull-Ups." The writer, Tara Parker-Pope, went on to explain that studies on women and men doing pull-ups indicated, after weeks of training, men were able to learn to do a pull-up, and sometimes many pull-ups. Women, meanwhile, lagged pathetically behind, couldn't seem to do a pull-up if it'd save their life. Why? "Men and women who can do them tend to have a combination of strength, low body fat and shorter stature. During training, because women have lower levels of testosterone, they typically develop less muscle than men," explained the study's author to Parker-Pope. "In addition, they can't lose as much fat. Men can conceivably get to 4 percent body fat; women typically bottom out at more than 10 percent."

So that's that, I thought. *I'm not skinny; I'm tall; I have arms like an orangutan. Pull-ups just aren't for me.* Anytime I thought of pull-ups, I thought also of that article, how completely confident in its conclusions it was. Who was I to defy science, research, experts?

But at the time, I had many kinds of strength I hadn't gotten to explore yet and was encountering just one of the many ways that research on strength was shortchanging women.

There is, overall, much less research on women and exercise than there is on men. For much of the time strength training has been studied, research has been conducted on men and then mapped onto women as if they were just smaller men with more biological complications, like menstruation. While this approach simplified things for researchers, coaches, and everyone in between, it tends to focus pityingly on all the ways women are worse at strength training than men: the fluctuating hormones; the relative lack of testosterone that encourages muscle growth; less lean muscle volume.

Testosterone, which tends to be higher in men, is famously the "muscle size–building hormone." The lack of it has long been taken as an indicator that women are inferior at strength or muscle building. But the more "female" hormone, estrogen, actually has protective qualities for muscle. We know because when estrogen starts to trend downward postmenopause, women tend to start losing muscle (as well as bone mass). One new study in 2022 found that one of the best ways to augment a decline in estrogen in order to protect muscle was—you guessed it—exercise. Women also tend to have higher levels of progesterone, which helps bodies process protein into new muscle fiber. It seems that, while stereotypically male hormones help muscles become bigger and stronger in the absolute, stereotypically female hormones help muscles heal faster and process protein more efficiently. Women's bodies may thus be better at preserving the muscle they get and more efficient at building the same amount of muscle with less effort.

When women's and men's strength are compared, and we put both groups in a study and find women are smaller and less strong than men, this also often happens without consideration of their training history (or related nutrition and recovery, which are equally as important as training). This is about as biased as science gets. Women's strength and muscle size are often compared unfavorably to men's, relative to their overall size and weight. But men are far more likely to have had exposure to sports and physical training than women, even as young kids. Even by the time the two groups are in high school, a boy is much more likely to have years of physical training under his belt and then spend sports practice time lifting weights. A woman who has been shortchanged on ever developing her strength, of course, won't be able to benefit as much from specific pull-up training as a man who is more likely to have trained before.

Most people will never learn to lift 400 or 600 or 1,000 pounds. But virtually everyone could learn to bench 95 pounds or deadlift 135 pounds, and genetic potential for strength and body composition for the two sexes are overlapping spectrums. Not every man is stronger than every woman, just as every man is not taller than every woman. A big reason that we believe women are "worse" at strength is the fact that "strength" is defined by what men do well, or are cultured to do well, versus what women can do better if given the chance.

Now that I was into strength training, pull-ups seemed to be everywhere, especially on social media. They were all the rage, the perfect way to show off athletic prowess. Men did them, and importantly, women also did them. But they weren't just for show, either: pull-ups were an important cornerstone of all lifting motion. Overhead vertical pulls balanced out the horizontal pulls, vertical pushes, and horizontal pushes. Pull-up work was frequently used in workout programs I saw, but the target audience for those programs was clearly those who could already do lots of pull-ups in one go. When I started lifting, I could barely grab on to the pull-up bar and manage a clench of my arm muscles before I had to let go and drop back down. This wasn't promising. But now, at least, I knew that Tara Parker-Pope might be wrong after all: just because this was my current reality, it was not my fate.

For a lift like the pull-up, where my body was the weight, how well I could execute had to do with my proportions relative to my strength. For a woman with about the same proportions as a man, a pull-up is no more out of reach for her than it is for him. So I started practicing, first with a pull-up machine where I rested my knees on a platform. I quickly learned that the machine messed with my ability to learn to move while I was hanging freely. I moved on to practicing "negatives"—jump up to the top of the pull-up bar, let myself down as slowly as possible—at the end of every workout. I tried to hold the negatives for as long as I could in sets of three, slowly counting to myself more and more seconds before my arms gave out. I practiced for months. While I couldn't gain much strength on my cut, the fact that I was slowly losing about ten pounds meant that my pull-ups would slowly get slightly easier on their own. After about six months had gone by, I was letting myself down during a twelve-second negative when I realized that that had become an absurdly long time. I dropped back down, tried to shake the exertion out of my arms, and looked up at the pull-up handles. This time I wouldn't be jumping up all the way—I'd be starting at the bottom.

I hopped up to grab the cracked plastic handles, swinging my feet back and forth a little to shift my weight and adjust my grip. Then I started to pull. Slowly, to my surprise, I rose up as the muscles in my back and arms clenched. As I got closer to the bar, I craned my chin, reaching to bring it over the top. My rise slowed and slowed, but I wasn't about to give up this close. I jerked at the bar and kicked my feet just a tiny bit—technically cheating, but I didn't come this far just to give up—and made it.

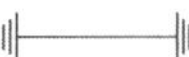

My cut started to slow down, and clothes that had become tight over the winter relaxed a little bit. But there were a few pieces where there was no going back. I tried on my fitted black stretchy work pants, the other half of my little road-tested work uniform. They were the pants I'd been wearing in a photo I'd shown my mom, the only time she'd expressed mild concern about my weight. I hadn't taken the picture with the goal of looking like anything, weight-wise; it was a cool photo, with the sunset behind me, and I'd been holding my new fixed-gear bike, standing in the middle of a Brooklyn street. "You look thin," she had said, not with admiration but with hesitation. Now the pants no longer accommodated my butt or legs.

After about twelve weeks of cutting, I'd lost ten pounds, and with it all of the indifference toward eating that I'd felt at the end of my bulk. I'd brought my calories down to 1,850 for the last few weeks as the effects of the deficit slowed down, and while I was still eating plenty of food, I missed snacks, cookies, french fries, chips. I missed ordering whatever at restaurants and having to opt for salads or the more restrained fish dishes, or having to make more of my own food because restaurants never gave you enough of whatever the protein was. Most of all, I missed crushing it in the gym, pushing for more reps and more weight. But now that I'd cut, I was all set up to bulk again, after a short maintenance period.

The day after a rest day, I woke up and made a fat stack of protein pancakes and laid a thick slice of butter on each one as they cooled on the counter. I opened the fridge, reached past the sugar-free maple syrup I'd learned about on YouTube, and grabbed the old-timey jug of grade A I'd bought at the grocery store the day before. I gave the pile a good drenching, then sat down with my coffee and dug in. Today was deadlift day.

30

The Final Test

AS I WRAPPED UP the end of my cut, I was also rapidly approaching my first powerlifting meet. I had moved to a new neighborhood in Brooklyn, which meant I had to leave Richie's behind, and I'd joined a new gym that was closer to where I lived. Called Murder of Crows Barbell Club, it was a massive, brick-walled, high-ceilinged former machine shop fronted by a garage. Plants grew through cracks in the mortar, and sunlight fell in through a trapdoor that led to the roof. In the winter it was freezing, and in the summer it was an oven. Where Richie's was a forest, Murder of Crows was an orderly little farm: nearly the entire floor was covered in lifting platforms, and on them stood one lifting rack after another. And though it was entirely targeted to lifters, it was more forthrightly welcoming of beginners.

While I'd come to love Richie's for all its quirks, Murder of Crows and its members seemed like they were created in a lab just for me. During the busiest hours, lifters sprawled across the green Astroturf running along one side, stretching and warming up, while everyone else hung off their equipment, clad in lifting belts and squat shoes. Members were incredibly polite about equipment, putting things away in their designated places as if it were an extra-fastidious preschool, or asking if anyone was using an item before they took it. Our own workout stuff, however, was scattered everywhere on the floor: belts, multiple pairs of shoes, chalk, straps, knee sleeves, energy-drink cans, water bottles. The gym offered programming that any member could follow and get coaching for. This allowed many of us to simultaneously suffer through and complain when we were all assigned the same exercises by the resident coach, Sean: seal rows; density rows; reverse barbell lunges; deadlift singles every minute, on the minute. The coaches played '90s alternative rock or rap on the gym's sound system. Members made faces or danced in the background of videos of one another's lifts, and some brought their dogs to hang out and receive pets while they lifted. There were as many women as men, and sometimes more. Many of the members were, like me, not good at all at lifting but took themselves as seriously as everyone else, which was often not seriously at all.

Whenever one member was about to start a heavy attempt, everyone would usually stop what they were doing to watch and scream "UP!" as the person fought through their lift. Once, a member named Mark stepped out of the rack with a barbell to squat it, knocking out one of the J-hooks as he did so, such that he wouldn't be able to put the bar back. As he did his reps, one of the other members, Lizzy, tried to help by maneuvering the fallen hook back into place, but she couldn't get the orientation right. She became flustered as the whole gym turned to watch while she helplessly bobbled the hook—Mark now standing there with the barbell on his back, waiting for her. She started to turn red and giggle. The rest of us started to giggle, too.

"Lizzy!" Mark yelled. Now he was trying not to laugh, because he was trying not to drop the 300-pound barbell.

Finally, she dropped the J-hook and squealed and stumbled away, weeping with laughter tears at how inept she was. Jean, who had been lifting since he was practically in diapers, stepped in and righted the hook easily, and Mark set the barbell down, drooping with exhaustion but letting out his held-in guffaws.

I hadn't been there long when people started asking me things like where the clips were, or if it was okay to use certain sets of plates. The interlopers and unsolicited-advice givers were not in residence, but now I found myself watching other lifters. One day, I watched Sanai bench across from where I was doing safety-bar squats. I could spot a million little problems: grip too narrow, elbows flared, shoulder blades flared, feet too wide, bar hitting too high on her chest. But she finished all her reps, then reracked the bar and stood up, seeming bashful. I caught her eye. "You're getting stronger!" I said.

"Yeah," she said. "I'm no good, though."

I waved a hand away. "What is 'good'? We're all learning."

She nodded.

Coach Sean came over to me. "Before your next set," he said, "your core is still getting kind of floppy. Try to tuck your ribs under, and take a whole breath and get set before you start every rep."

"Yes, Coach," I said. He had given me this feedback three dozen times before, but in his infinite patience, and for my sake, he pretended every time as if he were saying it for the first time. "Here I go, Coach."

Murder of Crows regularly held its own competitions, and members also traveled to competitions elsewhere. I'd come to understand competing in lifting as less of a sport for accomplished athletes and more like run-of-the-mill 5Ks or mud runs: people signed up to do them just to have a goal, not because they had any aspiration of winning. When I learned a bunch of members were going up to the Hudson Valley for the New York state championships, I signed up.

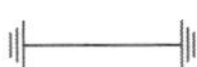

After three months of regimented training for the New York state meet, I arrived in the little upstate town via Metro-North, weighed down by multiple gym bags. I had done a water cut for this meet, meaning I was manipulating my food and water intake to just squeak into the weight class a few pounds below where I normally sat, since the next class up encompassed about twenty more pounds I didn't have as leverage. By the time I was walking through the subway station early in the morning to make it to the meet upstate, I was powerfully thirsty. I saw an abandoned half-full bottle of purple Gatorade and who-knew-what lying on the ground and felt a biological pull to pick it up and drink it. I arrived at the gym a few hours later, made my weigh-in, and began refueling with the little kit I'd brought along: a nice salty Cup Noodles, my own red Gatorade, plenty of water.

The meet weekend was divided up into shifts, so only women were lifting in the morning. They had arrayed themselves among the chairs set up for the audience, but as the meet time drew near, they moved their setups back to the warm-up area so the spectators could file in. I sat in a chair and braided my gym friend Leah's strawberry-blonde hair into two French braids on either side of her head.

With their lifting singlets on and looks of determination on their faces, women began pacing the warm-up area like tigers, with cool expressions and near-unblinking eyes. Family members or their handlers scuttled nervously around each of them, peppering them with questions or offering them various objects: a sports drink, a bag of candy, chalk for her hands, baby powder for her legs. The woman would either accept or briskly shake them off, without the usual beseeching eye contact that implored the other person not to be mad at her for whatever it was she wanted—any widening of her field of concern would break her concentration.

When called to the barbell by the meet announcer (who was, again, Geno, the goth pirate from the last meet I'd seen), each woman moved with powerful speed, not as a show of courage but because she'd been finally freed from waiting her turn. On squats, each woman gripped the bar and sized it up before ducking under and settling it on her shoulders, popping it out of the rack with a determined upward lift. On the bench, they approached the seat and, catlike, assumed an intricate process of contorting their upper body into an arch from butt to shoulders that would shorten the distance of travel for the barbell and optimize the lift, pressing their feet into place under their hips to drive their legs into the arch. On deadlifts, each woman hovered her face over the barbell before stomping one foot and then another into place right next to it, holding out her arms and hands over it as if casting a spell before tucking down to grab it and power it off the ground.

During every lift, their faces transformed into gorgeous grotesques, ranging in shape from merry Chinese parade dragons to Gothic gargoyles to Looney Tunes characters with steam coming out their ears. Sometimes they moved so fast they sent shock waves through their dangling braids and ponytails; sometimes they hung in the air for an astonishing number of seconds, with 300, 350, 400 pounds in their hands or on their back, turning redder as time seemed to stop until it suddenly sped up again and the woman was standing, her face returned to shape, and she was grinning with glee, undoing her belt with gusto while looking to the three lights that let the judges grade her lift. "Twenty-seven white lights" is considered a badge of honor to carry away from a powerlifting meet and stands for three white lights on all three attempts on all three lifts. If there were two or three red lights, most women set their mouths, shook their heads in a little frustration, and strode off the platform, ready to wait pent-up for the next attempt to prove the red lights wrong.

On each lift, every lifter gets three attempts, which are spent very strategically. The first lift is a "gimme," an amount of weight she could lift on the third day of a cold after her dog just died. The second is perhaps a tiny reach but mathematically pretty safe, still within her ability. The third is a leap of faith, well above any amount she has attempted before, but she's praying that the confluence of extra rest, extra food, extra adrenaline, and friends screaming her name will slingshot her beyond the realm of what she thought was possible.

I warmed up in the back of the room with my fellow lifters, testing my squats first with measured submax sets. When my name was called, I stepped out to the platform to cheers, and the crowd fell quiet as I set up, shouldered the barbell, and stepped out of the rack. "Squat!" said one of the judges, and I quickly dropped down before reversing motion while the crowd screamed "UP!" I did my first and second attempts easily, and for my third attempt, my coach entered a weight I'd never even touched before but was determined to try: 253 pounds, the equivalent of one red 25-kilogram and one blue 20-kilogram Eleiko plate loaded onto either end of the barbell. I returned to the warm-up area as I did after each attempt, but this time my stomach churned with nerves while I waited in the back to be called again. I looked at the other women around me. Some of them had finished with their squats and were beginning highly technical bench-press warm-ups, working with resistance bands. Others sat against the wall, giant headphones on, eyes closed, focusing or else meditating. One woman wept in the arms of her coach because she had thought she needed to wait at the bottom of her squat for the judges to command her to come back up and had failed her lift badly, paused for the command that was not coming.

As someone who becomes almost pathologically invested in anything that might be categorized as a distraction, I realized that I hadn't thought about virtually anything else except this meet in several days. The editor in chief who had recently hired me at our publication was rumored to be leaving for a new job. I was owed a text from a Tinder date.

Normally those things would send me into a spiral of constructing a narrative, theorizing about what everyone was thinking, what might happen next. Now they felt long ago and far away, as if they'd happened to someone in a fictional story. I had worked for months to peak for this meet, doing increasingly technical heavy reps, testing my attempts in the gym, resting up, eating my food, hydrating. It had all coalesced into this moment that might finally let me get 253 pounds up; the opportunity might not come again for months. I knew exactly what needed to happen this day, which meant I felt complete clarity about how inane and irrelevant everything else currently was.

When my name was called, I walked out to the platform, stepped up to the barbell, and grabbed it. Checking my hand placement before pulling myself under, I tucked it against the backsides of my shoulders and hoisted it out of the rack. I'd never felt weight this heavy before, and it swayed me like a skyscraper in a hurricane, my body's muscles doing a million little microadjustments per minute to stay under it and keep me from getting off-balance. I got still and looked up at the judge. "Squat," they said. My instinct was to dive-bomb at the ground immediately, but I paused with my gaze a few feet in front of me. I drew in a long breath and felt it fill up my core against my belt, then gripped my core muscles around it. Now I could start. The spotters on either side followed me down as the weight crunched my torso into my upper legs—I'd misgrooved, and my center of balance had now shifted dangerously forward. As I reversed out of the hole, the force of the rebound compounded the shift, and I tracked forward even more, straining to get the weight back on track as my heels peeled off the ground. My legs and head shook with effort as my rise ground to a halt for a beat. But I stopped only as if it were a required checkpoint; as soon as it was complete, I continued my way up until I was standing, balanced on my very tippy-toes, praying for the last command before I pitched forward and sent the barbell rolling off the back of my neck. "Rack," said the judge. I let out my breath and stepped one foot forward and then the other in rapid succession, catching the weight where it was trying to go before settling it back in the rack. I turned to the lights—three whites. I ran to Coach Sean and jumped on him and hugged him, who, though strong for his size, fought not to collapse under my weight.

Now it was time to bench. Bench had always been by far my most inconsistent lift, though it had gotten much better after I decided to simply bench every training day, for multiple sets, until it didn't scare me anymore. Still, any time I didn't eat or sleep enough, or it was that time of the month, my arms were the first to feel it. I was feeling all-powerful at the meet but knew I had a tendency to overestimate my bench, to want to force it to be better than it was through sheer determination, the equivalent of wearing shorts in order to force springtime to start. I pumped out my first attempt at 121 pounds no problem—it was a little shaky off my chest but otherwise smooth. The gossip of the warm-up area was that the judge was forcing everyone to pause the bar on their chest for an absurdly long time. This greatly compounded the difficulty of the lift; every second with a hundred-some pounds hovering over your chest feels like a lifetime. All that was technically needed was a stable touch, but the judge seemed to insist on the bar coming to a full, unequivocal, motionless stop before he'd give the command to press it back up.

On my second attempt at 132 pounds, I stuttered. After the eternity of a pause on my chest, I tried to reverse it up and got halfway, only for the bar to shake precipitously in midair, until I was finally able to force it up. Two white lights, one red light—a success, but only barely. I stepped out a third time and lay down on the bench, bending myself into an arch before pressing the barbell of 143 pounds up and out. "Start," said the judge.

I lowered the barbell down until it hit my chest. I waited, and waited, and waited. Did he fall asleep? "Press," he said.

I pressed, and almost before it even got started, the barbell fell back toward my sternum. Three red lights. The spotters tore the barbell out of my hands so fast that a judge lectured me for not holding on to it.

Finally, it was time for deadlifts. The volunteers carried away the big, unwieldy pieces of the competition rack, so that the platform held only the barbell and a simple jack. I instantly got nervous; not wanting to leave anything to chance in terms of drained energy from the first six attempts, I started chugging a twenty-ounce carbonated energy drink I'd brought with me. Then I started doing my warm-up sets, and as soon as I'd strapped on my belt, I realized my fatal mistake. For a while now, I'd noticed that if I ate or drank too close to doing deadlifts, the active digestion seemed to build up some kind of gas pressure in my stomach that would then push uncomfortably on my insides when I tried to brace. Usually, I was working out after work, before dinner, so it didn't come up often enough for me to really remember it was a problem. But I'd chugged the entire energy drink, and now all the built-up pressure was gurgling around inside of me. The carbonation made the pressure ten times worse. It was a problem, at the worst possible time, that I couldn't undo.

The only way I knew to mitigate the pain even a little was to take a breath and try to brace at the top of the lift before I bent down to pick the weight up, instead of bending down first, then bracing. But sometimes this resulted in a bad brace that allowed my back to pull all the way into a U-bend. And sometimes, this didn't work at all.

My first two attempts were weights I'd pulled quite a bit before—248 and then 264 pounds. On 264, my stomach roiled and bulged over my belt, putting huge pressure on the top of my stomach, but I stood up. As I walked back to my coach, he asked if I felt like I wanted to play it conservative with 275, or let it rip with 287. I'd never touched 287 before. But this was my last lift of the meet, my last chance to go big. I decided I'd rather die by 287 than live with 275. "Let it rip," I said.

"Let it rip?"

"Let it rip."

I stepped back into the warm-up area and wondered what exactly I was doing. What if my stomach literally burst open in front of everyone? What if I puked? My brain steered me through that detailed visual, and I shook it away. We are talking about a sport, and specifically a lift, where people fainted, peed on the platform, or left blood on the barbell with regularity. I'd never seen someone actually vomit. I hoped I'd realize the feeling before it actually happened, though my brain was so blank while lifting, always, that I couldn't be sure I'd be able to stop.

I was called back out and stepped to the loaded barbell. I snapped my belt closed, bent down, fluttered my fingers around the knurling, and hung there, looking at my feet, breathing in and out. *Which breath feels like it won't undo me? There, that one.* I held it down and crunched my core muscles around it, set my gaze in front of me, and started to power off the ground. Right away, the force of the breath crushed itself against my sphincter, and the pressure felt like it ricocheted right up into my face. The weight rose to above my knees; I was so close, but I felt about to pop. All of a sudden, I burped hollowly inside my mouth. The pressure disappeared. I felt a wave of emotional and physical relief, but my body continued through my lift as if nothing had happened. "Down," said the judge, and I dropped the barbell. Three white lights. I had lifted almost eight hundred pounds across my three best lifts. The crowd cheered and I ran back into the warm-up area, unclipping my belt and throwing it toward my pile of stuff with rapture. My legs and arms and back felt joyously hollow as I watched Leah and then Gaby pull deadlifts of well over three hundred pounds without effort, as if they were picking up a stick off the ground. The event had lasted more than three hours, but the constant motion had made it feel like no time had passed at all.

The meet would continue on for the rest of the day into the next, as the higher weight classes of women and then men cycled through to make their attempts. Before that, the judges would assemble the strongest women on little podiums to hand out medals for each weight class. I would have stayed, except I had to go lie down. It was barely noon, but the day was already getting hot as I waited on the platform for the train back down to New York. Once in my apartment, I dropped my gym bag at the door and turned on the AC in the living room—my apartment had four whole rooms now (including an illegal bedroom)—peeled off my lifting singlet and climbed into bed. I had already had some post-workout snacks to keep from falling dead asleep on the way home. But now I was able to unwrap and dig into my toasted everything bagel with lox, cream cheese, onion, tomato, and capers that I'd picked up on the way home. I cracked open my orange juice and took a sip of my terrible coffee loaded with cream and sugar; I didn't even know why I was drinking it. I was ready to fall asleep. Not exactly out of lack of energy, though I was as physically exhausted as I'd ever been. It was that I'd finally been everywhere it felt reasonable to go in my bodily journey; I had finally found like minds and support and acceptance. I also had a firm sense that there wasn't some preternaturally gifted athlete inside me waiting to leap out and achieve, which was the kind of pressure under which I'd done everything up until then. Instead, I was filled with a small, tender little seedling of this relationship with myself, with this movement, that mattered only to me and was only for me, and most importantly, I did not care for it to matter to anyone else.

I opened my laptop on my bed and hit Play on a movie. My cat jumped up and lay down with his weight against my right arm, vigorously lapping at the fur on the side of his stomach, now a little deflated with age. I knew no matter how much I ate I'd still wake up a little stiff and sore, but the food could only help. I curled up around my laptop and cat, surrounded by errant sesame and poppy seeds, and fell into a deep slumber.

31

Back to the Deadlift

IN ALL MY YEARS of lifting, I'd struggled on and off with deadlifts. No matter how I wanted to use my butt and hamstrings to lift the barbell, I couldn't consistently direct energy away from the small muscles of my lower back, which kept rounding out of its straight position. After a while, I started experimenting with "sumo" deadlifts, where my feet were straddled wide, both arms gripping the bar between my legs. Sumo deadlifts were more hip-centric, everyone said, which used the big muscles, like one's glutes, more and emphasized the lower back less. I was instantly in love with the way the more upright position seemed to remove my lower back from the equation almost entirely.

But about a year and a half into sumo deadlifting, I began to notice a problem. The upward motion seemed to tug painfully on the back and inside of my left leg. The heavier the weight was, the sharper the pain. I'd had lots of form issues and a lot of success working through them. But no matter how I tried to tweak my stance or movement pattern, the leg pain in the sumo position persisted. It was to the point that the barbell was starting to break from the floor unevenly on my heaviest weights, right side followed by left, and then it twisted in the air as I tried to force it up.

I asked Coach Sean for his input. "Yeah, you deadlift pretty much entirely with your inner hamstrings," he said. *Oh.* I was further from doing a proper sumo deadlift than I'd ever imagined.

In all four of my years of lifting, I had yet to experience a really meaningful setback. I'd had interruptions, been sick or gone on vacation or mooned over a breakup for slightly too long. But this was the first time that my body was seemingly lying down in the gains road and refusing to budge—or to give me any clear indication of what I could do to help it. All I wanted was to keep going down the path, getting stronger, doing my reps, recovering, and training again the next day. I'd been doing so without incident for a very long time. And now my leg was, without explanation, suddenly going to act up? And not only that, but act up worse the longer I tried to ignore it and pretend there was nothing wrong? I was overcome with the injustice of it—here I was, doing all that I could to take care of myself and get stronger, and my leg had the nerve, the gall, after all this time, to simply be like, *No thanks; I'd rather not*?

It filled me with dread to be literally hamstrung from going about my business. Lifting felt like the only pure, totally good, uncompromised thing I'd ever found in my life. What if I couldn't deadlift anymore? What if this injury radiated outward, and I wasn't even able to squat anymore? What if my days of glute-building exercises were over? No more lower-body days? No more quads?

I sought out a sports medicine doctor, who told me I had a mild hamstring strain and referred me to physical therapy.

My physical therapist, Sarah, was a woman easily half my size, clad in standard business casual. The physical therapy office was essentially a gym, equipped with various lifting machines, TRX straps, yoga mats, yoga balls, medicine balls, and giant spools of resistance band that the physical therapists could perfunctorily unwind, snip off, and tie into loops of appropriate length, like elves handling gift-wrap ribbon at the North Pole. I explained my injury to her and how it seemed to have happened, that I was a powerlifter and wanted to go back to powerlifting.

"We're going to try strengthening your other muscles, so they can take some pressure off of that one muscle that's strained," she said. Sarah got down on a yoga mat and had me anchor her ankles behind her as she kneeled facing away from me. Sarah was small and businesslike, but apparently under her sensible slacks and flats, she was built like a tank: she easily and slowly lowered her torso down to the floor by hinging at her knee joints, arms crossed across her chest, and then even snapped back up.

"You try," she said.

I assumed the position, knees on the floor with Sarah holding my ankles behind me. I tried to lean forward and control my motion but made it barely a couple of inches before my top half collapsed toward the ground. I caught myself on my hands just before my face smashed into the floor.

"Good! Again," Sarah said. Nothing seemed good about this. Theoretically, I lifted; why didn't I have any leg strength at all in this specific movement? I felt like a fawn taking its first steps. Sarah made me do ten reps, each more humiliating than the last. I pushed myself up on the last one, sweating, my face beet red.

She worked me through a few more movements, then set me up with a cold pack on my hamstring and handed me several printed sheets with a series of movements that would be my homework. It was everything I loathed about working out: three sets of ten reps of a bunch of different tiny movements, the very ones I'd come to hate from years of ineffective fitness-guru and women's-media workouts-lite. Clamshells. Side-lying hip abductions. Single-leg glute bridges. All on both sides. Almost two hundred reps of these twitchy exercises. Even though I had a full-time job, my insurance only covered a handful of PT sessions; the rest would come to more than $1,000 over eight weeks.

I'd rarely had to do more for any injury than just wait it out, or given much thought to the idea of having to actively rehabilitate or manage an injury. When I'd started to get intractable injuries from running, I just changed sports, in part because I was already fed up with running anyway. I didn't have this option with lifting.

"What should I do about my lifting workouts in the meantime?" I asked Sarah.

"You just don't want to push too hard right now. The first task is getting better."

As much as I wanted to thrash against this wisdom, she was right. I'd tried to push through and only made it worse.

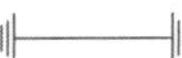

This was one of the first times I worried that I could have an injury that might never heal. I'd spent so long scoffing at lifting injuries I assumed were reserved for macho meatheads that I hadn't considered the possibility that I'd get injured, too, or how much of my relationship to lifting still rested on my being able to do it somewhat perfectly, always on my terms.

I clung to activities and people like a baby koala to its mother's back, in some cases even when they were hurting me—running, boyfriend, diets, work. It was without self-regard, with an impossible expectation to both fix and be fixed, save and be saved once and for all, setting myself up for eternal disappointment.

The first form of progress I learned in lifting was adding weight to my lifts a little at a time, always going steadily up. But soon I learned there were many more ways to advance—adding reps, shortening rest, slowing down or speeding up the movements, or breaking them down and drilling them in smaller pieces. Then there was the progress that was less objective—reps that simply felt better, looked stronger, were more stable.

And then, after a long time, I learned that progress was not always about going up, going harder, doing better. Trying to force an upward trajectory while temporarily injured could make that injury permanent. Sometimes progress was just acceptance—of a flaw, of a setback, of what I needed in that moment. Acceptance that a rep or a set or a workout, or a week or a month or a year, was perhaps not what I'd expected but exactly what it needed to be at that time. Progress could be about going backward, letting go. I wasn't a machine to be broken; I was an animal who could be bitten and then heal.

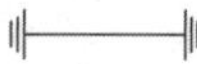

Every few sessions, Sarah gave me a new set of small accessory movements for homework: standing hip abductions, lunges, quadruped leg extensions. But the sessions at the office became increasingly intense. Many of the clients working out around me were being led gently through simple limb extensions or holding their balance on a stability mat while they picked up an object from the floor. But since Sarah knew I wanted to lift, she didn't hold back.

She kept running me through the humiliating Nordic leg curls, but also started working in single-leg squats while I held on to TRX straps (a move that was almost impossible for me); she set me up with a yoga ball on the floor that I lay in front of, face up. I rested one heel on the ball at a time, then performed a combo glute bridge, forcing my torso and butt up into the air, plus a hamstring curl to roll the ball underneath me with my heel, before rolling it back out again and repeating. She affixed a Velcro belt around my waist. Out of the belt was a curly bungee cord attached to the wall that Sarah had me try to bound away from in great, big leaps. I left every session pouring sweat.

Lifting had made me basically strong and more capable-feeling than ever, but once I started reaching out of that core mechanical comfort zone, there were still a lot of ways my body could move but wasn't really able to that made me collapse like a marionette. Yet, as with all the lifting I'd done, time plus effort plus enough shamelessness to accept being bad at it yielded results. The movements I was doing weren't weighted, but because I felt more aware of my body, I could feel myself getting a little better at them every time.

While I was having a better time than expected in PT, what wasn't really getting much better was my sumo deadlift. Every once in a while in the gym, against my better judgment, I'd get impatient and give it a shot again. And every time, my hamstring would fire up too hard. The pain was lessened, but I could still feel it coming alive in a way that wasn't entirely good. I was too afraid of what might happen if I tried my luck with the heaviest weights that I could do, so I didn't even venture into that range. Where I didn't experience pain was doing conventional deadlifts with my feet together. I started mixing them into my workouts, happy to be able to lift some weight without risking the dreaded twinge.

I asked Coach Sean what I should do. "Honestly," Sean said, "go back to conventional. Sumo is kinda overrated."

I hadn't thought of it that way. For everything sumo supposedly had going for it in general, it was hurting me specifically. After all that, I was hesitant to have to just give it up anyway. But conventional deadlifts, while they hadn't exactly clicked, hadn't committed the same offense.

Still, they were no picnic. With my hamstring problem now healed and solved, I could get a decent amount of weight up, but even small variations in form seemed to affect how sore my lower back would be the next day. Sean seemed at a loss for what might help.

When the pandemic rolled around, every gym closed and heavy weights were ripped out of my hands. I improvised with what I had at home—a 15-pound dumbbell, bags I could fill with heavy books or cast-iron pans, a planter I could fill up with water. By this time, I had a sense that I had one much weaker hip, on my left side. Why, exactly, was a mystery; it could be that it was the hip I didn't rest my weight on when I sat in a chair, or the hip that folded under when I played field hockey in high school and had to lean to the left side, as a lefty, to hit the little ball with my little stick.

I'd been throwing myself against the wall of heavy deadlifts, unwilling to back the weight down. But the pandemic forced my hand: with small weights, technique was all there was. I started working on my hip-hinging motion specifically, using the muscles in my hips and posterior chain to suspend the upper half of my body and stabilize against weight that might pull me forward.

I started drilling single-leg movements that targeted my hips individually: single-leg Romanian deadlifts, lunges, lateral step-ups. I still resented the chore of these little movements and often avoided working out entirely because modified home workouts felt like tedious wastes of time. But if I avoided working out for more than a few days, I tossed and turned in my sleep, went to bed too late, and woke up too early. Most weeks, I chided myself into a few workouts.

About eight months into the pandemic, November 2020, I was finally able to get my hands on some of my own weights at home and set them up on the patio in my tiny Brooklyn backyard. I charged back up through 95 pounds, 135 pounds, 155, 175, 205, 225, 255 on my deadlifts, ecstatic to be able to really lift again but even more ecstatic to find my form remained solid. The barbell got so heavy the plates started punching holes in the patio concrete. But I kept doing my accessory movements, too.

The next December, I decided to pull all my efforts together and attempt a 300-pound deadlift. In the past, very heavy deadlifts had always left me with aching lower back muscles, sometimes for days. Contrary to before the pandemic, my deadlifts had been feeling better and better. I did more deadlift reps and weight than ever before, and magically, the soreness started to burn in my glutes and my hamstrings, while my lower back remained at peace. Something in there had changed in all those months without my heavy weights.

But it's in the most intense range of weights where form is really put to the test. Where 275 pounds might not pull my nice, straight back out of shape, a 300-pound deadlift could.

I rested for three days leading up to my planned deadlift day, not wanting to take any chances on fatigue. When the day came, I warmed up carefully: 135 pounds, 185, 240, 270. As I set up in front of the 300-pound loaded barbell, my heart beat so loudly it felt as if it were echoing through the bare December trees contained on all sides by the buildings of our block. There were absolutely no stakes to this pull; if I failed it, no one would know or care except me. Still, by that time I hadn't faced a meaningful PR in almost four years, and really heavy deadlifts had always gotten the best of me. What if all the time and effort had meant nothing, and I'd been fooling myself?

I wiggled my fingers over the bar and toes under the bar, a strange habit I am barely conscious of but that my extremities seem to do on their own, as if they are casting some sort of jazz-hands incantation. I bent down to grip it, tilted my head up to set my gaze just a few feet in front of me, and pulled. The bar didn't drift or tilt. My back remained flat, my spine suspended straight as a rod from my hips, which hinged the bar steadily upward. I could feel my legs trembling a little with the effort, but they weren't giving in. I stood all the way up as I let out a victorious grunt before I dropped it back down to the patio, sending yet another crack zigzagging through the concrete, but I didn't care, because I finally deadlifted three hundred pounds. I could pick up the weight of my frailest, eating-disordered self and my bulkiest strong self, both at the same time.

Epilogue

IN THE SPRING OF 2022, to get a break from our tiny pandemic apartment, I moved temporarily to Joshua Tree with my boyfriend. I'd met him about four years after I started lifting and one year after beginning therapy to try and understand how to start letting go and trying not to control so much in the rest of my life, an unfortunate front seat for him to be sitting in. But he had a Midwestern ease and gentleness impressed upon him by his parents, and he understood because he was as searchingly introspective as I was: we were just two tall, silly jocks preoccupied with how to be. The most recent media company I worked for (staggering under, among other pressures, a significant amount of semisecret debt to Saudi Arabia and a failure to go public, later leading it to file for bankruptcy) had laid me off the previous year. So I started a newsletter where I wrote about strength and lifting weights, among other things. It did well enough that I didn't need another job. The competition was not stiff, but I was by far the best boss I'd ever had.

The temperature in Joshua Tree cracked 105 degrees most days we stayed there, with not a cloud in the sky. Stepping outside was like stepping into a sauna, which appealed to me deeply (always too cheap to join a fancy gym, but I love a good sweat).

I tried a bunch of gyms around town before joining one with a shabby deadlift platform, mismatched plates, and grubby, hideous yellow-and-red plastic flooring. The staff played chicken with the AC, trying to keep it only as cool as prevented most people from complaining. I did my deadlifts and squats, played around with their mountain-climber treadmill, and used the kickback and hip-thrust machines to really give my glutes what for. I had no idea how much I weighed.

The shabbiness of the gym reminded me spiritually of Richie's, where my whole journey had started. When I went to check up on their location online, I found the gym had closed in the pandemic and never reopened, but recent Google Map photos showed the signs outside were still intact. This suggested the crowded collection of equipment still sat inside, no longer getting the stuffing loved out of it by its clientele, gathering more dust, a many-limbed beast waiting to be awakened.

One day, I was driving along the Twentynine Palms Highway to seek out a hike. We were near a national park, and most of the surrounding area was vast, pin-drop-silent desert. The dirt and sand were interrupted here and there by mountains. High desert mountains were not mountains as I'd always understood them, the rounded bald heads and knees that bulged out of the upstate New York landscape. These were fresh and young piles of rocks. There were even stacks of boulders—huge, improbably shaped, unstable-looking boulders balanced just so on top of smaller ones, like a giant child's brief amusement before they ran off.

I pulled up to a hiking location I'd found online called Rattlesnake Canyon, expecting to find the usual dirt-and-sand trail winding its way up some kind of incline. But I didn't see one. I checked the trail reviews on an app. "Didn't get very far before we had to turn around. Looked cool for the parts we saw though," said one review of the trail. "Also, there isn't really a trail."

I followed a little path through some tall, wizened desert scrub toward the center of the canyon. The path quickly came to an end where the tumbling piles of rocks began. It then led up to a massive mountainside that rose sharply into the sky, littered with monzogranite boulders in speckled gray, white, and terra-cotta. I climbed on top of the first boulder, then started hopping from rock to neighboring rock. When I came to a space, I jumped down, then ran to the next boulder, an even bigger one, and launched myself onto it like a flying squirrel. With a pair of decently grippy shoes on the rough cuboid-textured surfaces, I was free to climb as high and as far as I could see; I was limited only by how much water I could carry.

I would not have thought that this more-than-hiking, less-than-rock-climbing would have done anything for me. But rock scrambling exists in the gap between hiking and fully equipped rock climbing. It's basically free climbing over, up, down, and between big boulders. As I climbed higher and farther, old instincts leapt out of me for grabbing here, shifting there, getting a toehold on this side to launch myself upward. My hips and legs were so strong, flexible, and independently stable that I could practically fly over and up the boulders. I felt more entirely myself than I had felt in a long, long time. To be outside, in the sun, scrambling over surfaces, stopping to crouch down and watch a California side-blotched lizard pause in his skitter between two crevices to watch me back.

I began going out rock scrambling regularly. The temperature would reach ninety degrees by 10 a.m., so I started to take off in the car as early as I could get out of the house to climb for a couple of hours. The lack of paths made for occasional slow going. I might pick a target high up and try to game out a route, only to find once I got a different angle on the boulders that it would not be so easy. It might be much steeper than I realized, or two of the boulders might be much farther apart than they had seemed from far away and, in fact, separated by a sheer ten-foot drop into a shadowy crevice. Then I'd have to back down out of the route and find another way. But it was okay; the act of climbing, the puzzling out of the surfaces as they unfolded, was the point. When I did manage to reach a vantage point, I'd sit down in some shade, if I could, and slurp from my little hydration fanny pack. Every time I left the canyon, I would be beet red, hair plastered to my face and neck, and I'd be eagerly anticipating the next time I would go back.

Epilogue

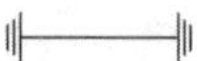

When my mom came to visit Joshua Tree, I decided to take her to Rattlesnake Canyon. I was slightly worried; at sixty-five, she was still active, mostly from long hours spent chasing my nephews around. Her knees had gotten bad enough that she had given up jogging, her lifelong cardio of choice. But she was excited to try it, so we went.

We drove out to the craggy edge of Joshua Tree National Park, pulled up to the canyon, and started climbing. My mom had brought her hiking boots, so her feet gripped the rough surface of the boulders as well as mine did. I had been impressed with myself when I'd started scrambling, surprised by how much skill I'd maintained from climbing all over every tree and play structure I could find as a kid. As we climbed, I noticed my mom had as many of these same instincts. But she was also braver than I was. A couple of times we came to some crevices between boulders, and while I would hesitate, sizing up the gap and mentally rehearsing how I'd pace my steps to lead up to my jump, she would simply hop across.

I remembered the hikes she used to take us on when all of us were kids, trekking up a steep hill in the woods in single file. Our feet would slip in the rich, decaying mush of old leaves and sticks, but if we were lucky, our mom was leading us to the top of a mountain with an old fire tower. We'd climb it as it swayed in the wind and look out on the endlessly rolling blue-green hills all around. If we were really lucky, she'd be leading us to a whole lake embedded in the top of the mountain, rippled by breezes and birds. She'd point out to us the giant rocks that were next to deep water so that we could jump off over and over again, trying to outdo each other with jackknifes, cannonballs, belly flops, flips, barrel rolls, until we were threatened with the onset of nighttime.

Unlike the tumbling stream of rocks that made up most of the canyon, the pile of rocks we were climbing looked like they had emerged volcanically from the earth at some point and dried into roughly two tiers, like a wedding cake. At the point where the tiers met, our path had led us to the biggest gap so far. We were standing on a tall, oblong rock with a sheer drop-off on all sides. Across a gap of several feet was the next rock, only about a foot wide, just under the upper tier. I peered down into the darkness of the crevice and got an overly realistic flash of missing the jump and then bouncing off the rough walls of the two rocks like a pinball, limbs contorted at all angles, until I landed crumpled on the bottom. I hesitated as the movie played back behind my eyes. While this happened, my mom jumped. My heart jumped, too, but it didn't even have time for a full leap before she landed safely on the other side, pressing her weight up against the wall and shimmying around to a wider outcropping. "Whoa," I said. "Be careful."

"I'm okay," she said.

I looked at the gap. "It feels far," I said, staring down in it again.

"You can do it," she said. I looked up at her, then back down at the gaping chasm, then again at the ledge. I took a deep breath and then another one. I felt the sensory memory of all the distant times I'd been betrayed by my body, when I felt like I was slipping through its cracks, and then all the more recent times it had caught me again and again. My core grabbed on to the next breath, I cocked my hips, and I jumped.

I landed hard on one foot, dragging the other gently behind it as I clung to the wall for dear life. I froze for a moment to absorb that nothing bad had happened. It hadn't been that far after all.

We wound around and around a pile of rocks until we were able to approach the peak from one side. My mom scrambled up to the top and sat down in a little indentation facing out over the expanse.

"You're doing great at climbing. I'm surprised," I said to my mom. "I mean, I was surprised for myself, too, that I seemed to remember so much from climbing when we were little. You have the instincts for it, too."

"Yeah, we played a lot," she said. "But you know, I've also been going to the gym."

I turned to her, hoping to not say the wrong thing. "Have you been lifting?"

"Not like you do. I do, you know, my squats with the smaller barbells. And my planks and my sit-ups."

"Oh, Mom," I said, smiling, turning back to the view. "Well, that's good. I'm glad for you."

We looked out over the expanse that sloped gently down toward the beginnings of the nearby military town. The flat landscape meant that sound traveled incredibly far, but I couldn't hear anything except the hot wind blowing in from the west as the sun intensified. It hadn't rained in many months, and the serpentine rock beds that had filled with spring runoff were now dry. But despite the intense sun and lack of water and soil, the boulder faces were pocked with desert bushes that had forced their roots down, into and between the rocks. They thrashed gamely in the burning breeze.

Before long, it would be time to climb back down, which I'd found could be even harder than the journey up. Instead of gravity working against me and tempering my speed, it would be trying to amplify my every movement. But the easiest way down was to embrace those brief and tiny losses of control, to stop fighting them and just let myself fall.

Author's Note

IN ORDER TO MAINTAIN anonymity, some names and identifying details of people and places have been changed. I have tried to recreate events, locales, and conversations from my memories, personal records, and historical records. Some of the content in this book draws from past work I have done writing for The Hairpin, *SELF*, *VICE*, and my own newsletter, *She's A Beast*.

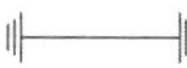

In this book, I make occasional reference to "women" and "men." But some of the references serve to explain how these are not two discrete groups with predictable respective traits. Sex and gender are spectrums—ones with peaks and valleys, but spectrums nonetheless. People with vaginas may find some science applies to them more than science developed with people with penises in mind; people with very different genetics than me may find some of the practices in this book affect them differently than they did me. But the most important takeaway here is that exercise, and especially lifting weights, is for everyone, regardless of their hormonal profile, height, weight, age, or anything else. It makes no more sense to gatekeep lifting weights based on these personal details than to prohibit use of a computer, driving a car, or having a job on this basis. (I know they've tried gatekeeping all those in the past, and thank God, none of them worked out.)

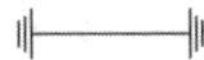

Finally, this book is not intended as a substitute for the medical advice of physicians. My life is not your life, my numbers are not your numbers, my story is not your story, and these things matter when it comes to health and biology. You should consult a physician on these issues relating to your health, particularly with respect to symptoms that may impact exercise or diet.

The information in this book is presented for entertainment and education and is not meant to supplement or replace proper strength training or dietary advice. Like any sport involving equipment, physical facility, and environmental factors, strength training poses some inherent risk. I and the publisher advise you to take full responsibility for your safety and know your limits. Do not take risks beyond your level of experience, aptitude, training, and comfort level.

Although I and the publisher have made every effort to ensure that the information in this book was correct at press time, we do not assume and hereby disclaim any liability to any party for any loss, damage, or disruption caused by errors or omissions, whether such errors or omissions result from negligence, accident, or any other cause.

Acknowledgments

A HUGE THANK YOU to the team at Grand Central Publishing for standing behind this book with two feet and giving it the lift (!) it needed: Staci Burt, Alana Spendley, Kristin Nappier, Ian Dorset. To my agent Anna Sproul-Latimer, I wish for your fairy-godmother-like advocacy for many more books to come. To John Timmer, who took me under his wing in my earliest days and taught me the ropes of good science reporting. To Kelsey McKinney, Jami Attenberg, Megan Greenwell, Josh Gondelman, and Katie Heaney, who all provided wonderful and sage counsel and/or much-needed companionship during the development of this book. To Georgia Cloepfil, whose assistance was invaluable during my early days of research. To Charlotte Markey, Chantal Gil, Sarah Riley, and Linda Rodriguez McRobbie, whose expertise and conversations with me provided a sounding board for these ideas.

Thank you to my readers, some of whom persist from my tech-reporting past to the present, and many of whom make the She's A Beast community the good-hearted, generous, and welcoming place it is. To the members of Richie's Bushwick, may it rest, and especially to Dimitrios. To the members and coaches of Murder of Crows Barbell. To anyone who has given *LIFT-OFF: Couch to Barbell* a shot, you are brave and I'm so proud of you.

Acknowledgments

A giant thank you to my editor, Karyn Marcus, who was bought into this project from day one and never wavered even while others did. Your careful, patient, and compassionate eye made this book what it is.

To my mother and siblings: You all have more courage than you know and thank you for putting up with me all these years.

Last but not least, to Seamus, for helping the growing menagerie continue to blossom, for always wanting to chat, and for never failing to make me laugh.

Notes

CHAPTER 3

14 **a user named Montereyo had posted her six-month weight-lifting progress:** Montereyo (u/montereyo), "6 month progress weightlifting (female)," Reddit, December 28, 2011, https://www.reddit.com/r/Fitness/comments/nue8c/6_month_progress_weightlifting_female/.

17 **"I lift to be strong":** Montereyo (u/montereyo), "6 month progress weightlifting (female)," Reddit, December 28, 2011, https://www.reddit.com/r/Fitness/comments/nue8c/comment/c3c1wn4/?utm_source=reddit&utm_medium=web2x&context=3.

CHAPTER 4

21 **"are you dieting too?":** Montereyo (u/montereyo). "6 month progress weightlifting (female)," Reddit, December 28, 2011, https://www.reddit.com/r/Fitness/comments/nue8c/comment/c3c0o2g/?utm_source=reddit&utm_medium=web2x&context=3.

21 **"I am not dieting, as in, actively trying to lose weight":** Montereyo (u/montereyo), "6 month progress weightlifting (female)," Reddit, December 28, 2011, https://www.reddit.com/r/Fitness/comments/nue8c/comment/c3c0o2g/?utm_source=reddit&utm_medium=web2x&context=3.

CHAPTER 5

32 **anywhere from 250 to 1,000, as various celebrities including Britney Spears:** Lara Walsh, "I Worked Out Like Britney Spears for a Week and My Abs Have Never

Felt So Sore," Business Insider, October 29, 2019, https://www.businessinsider.com/i-worked-out-like-britney-spears-for-a-week-how-2019-10.

32 **and Lindsay Lohan:** Amanda Fortini, "Lindsay Lohan as Marilyn Monroe in 'The Last Sitting,'" *New York Magazine*, February 15, 2008, https://media.nymag.com/fashion/08/spring/44247/.

32 **Much is made of "core" strength:** Mark Rippetoe, *Starting Strength* (Wichita Falls: Aasgaard Company, 2011), 18, Kindle.

CHAPTER 8

52 **freeing up that hot, fast energy:** Chris Camacho et al., *Certified Personal Trainer*, 7th ed. (National Academy of Sports Medicine, 2024), chap. 8, NASM.org.

55 **without the complex web of macro- and micronutrients:** William J. Kraemer and Nicholas A. Ratamess, "Hormonal Responses and Adaptations to Resistance Exercise and Training," *Sports Medicine* 35, no. 4 (2005): 339–61, https://doi.org/10.2165/00007256-200535040-00004.

55 **everything gets put to use properly:** G. Greogry Haff and N. Travis Triplett, *Essential Principles of Strength Training*, 4th ed. (Champaign, IL: Human Kinetics, 2016), 94.

CHAPTER 9

62 **when they go back to eating:** Jennifer L. Gaudiani, *Sick Enough: A Guide to the Medical Complications of Eating Disorders* (New York: Taylor & Francis, 2019), 78, Kindle.

62 **makes us deeply mentally unwell:** Jennifer L. Gaudiani, *Sick Enough: A Guide to the Medical Complications of Eating Disorders* (New York: Taylor & Francis, 2019), 23–24, Kindle.

62 **our senses become blunted:** Allison Whitten, "The Brain Has a 'Low-Power Mode' That Blunts Our Senses," *Quanta Magazine*, June 14, 2022, https://www.quantamagazine.org/the-brain-has-a-low-power-mode-that-blunts-our-senses-20220614.

62 **even paranoid, about following rules:** Ancel Keys et al., *The Biology of Human Starvation*, vol. 1 (Minneapolis: University of Minnesota Press, 1950).

62 **lack of food quality and nutrient balance—contributes to cravings:** Sushil Sharma et al., "Psychology of Craving," *Open Journal of Medical Psychology* 3, no. 2 (2014): 120–25, https://doi.org/10.4236/ojmp.2014.32015.

63 **malnutrition then feeds into an increase in addictive behaviors, even substance abuse:** Asia Afzal et al., "Nutrition and Substance-Use Disorder," in *Nutrition and Psychiatric Disorders*, ed. Wael Mohamed and Firas Kobeissy, Nutritional Neurosciences (Singapore: Springer, 2022), 289–312, https://doi.org/10.1007/978-981-19-5021-6_14.

63 **misread hunger cue for protein:** Tim Vernimmen, "Like Hungry Locusts, Humans Can Easily Be Tricked into Overeating," *Knowable Magazine*, May 1, 2023, https://doi.org/10.1146/knowable-050123-1.

63 **call these snacks "protein decoys":** Tim Vernimmen, "Like Hungry Locusts, Humans Can Easily Be Tricked into Overeating," *Knowable Magazine*, May 1, 2023, https://doi.org/10.1146/knowable-050123-1.

CHAPTER 10

67 **African mango seeds would make me lose ten pounds:** Jim Chiang, "Dr. Oz Recent Affirmation That African Mango Is an Effective Weight Loss Supplement Coincides with New Supplement from Bel Marra Nutritionals," PRWeb, December 17, 2011, https://web.archive.org/web/20120209161335/https://www.prweb.com/releases/2011/12/prweb9049112.htm.

67 **a survey of four thousand of its readers on their eating habits:** Tula Karras, "The Disorder Next Door," *SELF*, May 2008, 248.

68 **what is now called "atypical" anorexia:** Megen Vo et al., "Medical Complications and Management of Atypical Anorexia Nervosa," *Journal of Eating Disorders* 10 (2022): 196, https://doi.org/10.1186/s40337-022-00720-9.

68 **more than three times as many people have atypical anorexia versus "typical" anorexia:** Erin N. Harrop et al., "Restrictive Eating Disorders in Higher Weight Persons: A Systematic Review of Atypical Anorexia Nervosa Prevalence and Consecutive Admission Literature," *International Journal of Eating Disorders* 54, no. 8 (2021): 1328–57, https://doi.org/10.1002/eat.23519.

70 **steer their way back to an existence of "gentle nutrition":** Evelyn Tribole and Elyse Resch, *Intuitive Eating: A Revolutionary Anti-Diet Approach*, 4th ed. (New York: St. Martin's Press, 2020), 229, Kindle.

71 **has 25 grams of protein:** "Chicken and Turkey Nutrition Facts," United States Department of Agriculture Food Safety and Inspection Service, September 2011, https://www.fsis.usda.gov/sites/default/files/media_file/2020-10/Chicken_Turkey_Nutrition_Facts.pdf.

CHAPTER 11

80 **may induce the creation of new neurons and new memories:** Bente Klarlund Pedersen, "Physical Activity and Muscle–Brain Crosstalk," *Nature Reviews Endocrinology* 15, no. 7 (2019): 383–9, https://doi.org/10.1038/s41574-019-0174-x.

CHAPTER 12

86 **Women tend to have between 7 and 23 percent:** Carsten Roepstorff et al., "Higher Skeletal Muscle a_2AMPKActivation and Lower Energy Charge and Fat Oxidation in Men Than in Women During Submaximal Exercise," *Journal of Physiology* 574, no. 1 (2006): 125–38, https://doi.org/10.1113/jphysiol.2006.108720.

86 **more type I muscle fibers than men:** James L. Nuzzo, "Sex Differences in Skeletal Muscle Fiber Types: A Meta-Analysis," *Clinical Anatomy* 37, no. 1 (2023): https://doi.org/10.1002/ca.24091.

CHAPTER 14

100 **nothing but squatting for three months:** Megan Gallagher (megsquats), "Road to 300# Squat," YouTube, October 7, 2014, https://www.youtube.com/watch?v=YC5WuW5cNIQ.

100 **"I really hated it, I hated it so bad":** Megan Gallagher (megsquats), "My Fitness Journey and Body Transformation(s): Couch to Bikini to Powerlifter," YouTube, April 3, 2015, https://www.youtube.com/watch?v=EXmfQ6F04wU.

CHAPTER 15

103 **"My strength numbers shot upward":** Daniel Duane, "How the Other Half Lifts: What Your Workout Says About Your Social Class," *Pacific Standard*, July 23, 2014, https://psmag.com/social-justice/half-lifts-workout-says-social-class-85221.

104 **"She's just a gag character whose humor stems from being the opposite of a hot exotic chick":** "Brawn Hilda," TVTropes, May 27, 2010, https://tvtropes.org/pmwiki/pmwiki.php/Main/BrawnHilda.

104 **Big Rhonda from *That '70s Show*:** Technically, Big Rhonda is classified as a "huge schoolgirl" on TV Tropes; while those literal words aren't untrue, I dispute this classification. "That '70s Show," TV Tropes, accessed October 8, 2024, https://tvtropes.org/pmwiki/pmwiki.php/Series/That70sShow.

106 **with awards around culturally German holidays:** William J. Baker, *Sports in the Western World* (Totowa, NJ: Rowman & Littlefield, 1982), 101–2.

106 **Jahn published *A Treatise on Gymnasticks*:** Friedrich Ludwig Jahn, *A Treatise on Gymnasticks* (Northampton, MA: S. Butler, 1828), https://archive.org/details/atreatiseongymn00jahngoog/page/n24/mode/2up.

106 **also for "controversial" causes, including abolition and socialism:** "Turnverein Movement [Turner Hall]," Texas State Historical Association, July 11, 2022, https://www.tshaonline.org/handbook/entries/turnverein-movement.

106 **on the basis of skin color, gender, or place of birth:** Annette Hofmann, *American Turner Movement: A History from Its Beginning to 2000*, trans. Ernestine Dillon et al.

(Indianapolis: Max Kade German-American Center at IUPUI and the Indiana German Heritage Society, 2010), 18, Kindle.

106 **using religious phrases on government currency or documents:** Annette Hofmann, *American Turner Movement: A History from Its Beginning to 2000*, trans. Ernestine Dillon et al. (Indianapolis, Max Kade German-American Center at IUPUI and the Indiana German Heritage Society, 2010), 124, Kindle.

107 **and discouraged actual, equitable physical education:** Annette Hofmann, *American Turner Movement: A History from Its Beginning to 2000*, trans. Ernestine Dillon et al. (Indianapolis: Max Kade German-American Center at IUPUI and the Indiana German Heritage Society, 2010), 152, Kindle.

107 **Turners repeatedly served as Lincoln's bodyguards, including during his inauguration:** Annette Hofmann, *American Turner Movement: A History from Its Beginning to 2000*, trans. Ernestine Dillon et al. (Indianapolis: Max Kade German-American Center at IUPUI and the Indiana German Heritage Society, 2010), 110, Kindle.

107 **Turner clubs grew into a meeting place for working-class immigrants:** Annette Hofmann, *American Turner Movement: A History from Its Beginning to 2000*, trans. Ernestine Dillon et al. (Indianapolis: Max Kade German-American Center at IUPUI and the Indiana German Heritage Society, 2010), 17, Kindle.

107 **Spies was the editor of a radical labor-driven newspaper, a union supporter, and a Turner:** Annette Hofmann, *American Turner Movement: A History from Its Beginning to 2000*, trans. Ernestine Dillon et al. (Indianapolis: Max Kade German-American Center at IUPUI and the Indiana German Heritage Society, 2010), 17, Kindle.

107 **their duty to protect the less powerful and raise the floor for every person:** Devin Thomas O'Shea, "Socialist Gym Rats Fought to End Slavery in America," *Jacobin*, August 9, 2023, https://jacobin.com/2023/08/german-forty-eighters-immigrants-turners-exercise-socialists-abolitionists-civil-war/.

CHAPTER 16

112 **using a woman dressed in a Hooters uniform was a bit much:** Anita Sarkeesian (Feminist Frequency), "Women as Background Decoration: Part 1—Tropes vs Women in Video Games," June 16, 2014, https://feministfrequency.com/video/women-as-background-decoration-tropes-vs-women.

CHAPTER 18

121 **that their congregations had developed a manliness problem:** Brett McKay and Kate McKay, "When Christianity Was Muscular," The Art of Manliness, September 13, 2016, https://www.artofmanliness.com/character/knowledge-of-men/when-christianity-was-muscular/.

121 **how to talk about books and art and other "civilized" topics:** Brett McKay and Kate McKay, "When Christianity Was Muscular," The Art of Manliness, September

13, 2016, https://www.artofmanliness.com/character/knowledge-of-men/when-christianity-was-muscular/.

121 **no one to protect the United States from a growing threat of oversentimentality:** Clay Risen, *The Crowded Hour: Theodore Roosevelt, the Rough Riders, and the Dawn of the American Century* (New York: Scribner, 2019), 24, Google Books, https://www.google.com/books/edition/The_Crowded_Hour/s7GWDwAAQBAJ.

121 **because it would cause the development of "parasitic muscles":** Jason P. Shurley et al., *Strength Coaching in America,* Terry and Jan Todd Series on Physical Culture and Sports (Austin: University of Texas Press, 2019), 16, Kindle.

122 **neurasthenia was a new, wide-ranging diagnosis meant to capture "all the forms of and types of exhaustion coming from the brain":** Anson Rabinbach, *The Human Motor* (Berkeley: University of California Press, 1992), 153.

122 **"the performance of physiological functions is a source of generally painful sensations":** Emile Durkheim, *Suicide* (New York: The Free Press, 1979), 68.

123 **"which you speak of as standing in the way of perfect sanctification":** Charles G. Finney, *Lectures to Professing Christians* (E.J. Goodrich, 1879), "Christian Perfection—1," https://archive.org/details/lecturestoprofes00finn.

123 **"a power can be brought to bear against the kingdom of evil in the world by right body keeping":** James C. Whorton, *Crusaders for Fitness* (Princeton, NJ: Princeton University Press, 1982), 289–90.

123 **God also loved teamwork, cooperation, loyalty, and respect for authority:** Paul Putz, "Muscular Christianity and Moral Formation Through Sports," *Faith & Sports*, January 31, 2022, https://blogs.baylor.edu/faithsports/2022/01/31/muscular-christianity-and-moral-formation-through-sports/.

124 **it started to include physical recreation programming for all YMCAs in 1864:** William J. Baker, *Sports in the Western World* (Totowa, NJ: Rowman & Littlefield, 1982), 165.

124 **there were nearly four hundred YMCA gyms in the United States:** William J. Baker, *Sports in the Western World* (Totowa, NJ: Rowman & Littlefield, 1982), 165.

124 **a YMCA staffer coined the term "body building":** "1800–1899," YMCA, ymca.org, https://www.ymca.org/who-we-are/our-history/founding-years.

124 **"vitality and health essential to the success and happiness of life":** Bernarr Macfadden, "The Editor's Belief," *Physical Culture* 1 (1900): 7, https://hdl.handle.net/2027/umn.31951000756765k?urlappend=%3Bseq=7.

125 **in the form of government-sponsored fitness campaigns:** Conor Heffernan, "Fascist Physical Culture in 1930s Germany," Physical Culture Study, August 9, 2019, https://physicalculturestudy.com/2019/08/09/fascist-physical-culture-in-1930s-germany/.

125 **work out like fascists did in Germany and Italy:** Charlotte MacDonald, *Strong, Beautiful and Modern* (Vancouver, BC: UBC Press, 2011), 14.

125 **squat jumps, sit-ups, pull-ups, push-ups, and a three-hundred-yard run:** Brett McKay and Kate McKay, "Are You as Fit as a World War II GI?," The Art of

Manliness, September 12, 2011, https://www.artofmanliness.com/health-fitness/fitness/are-you-as-fit-as-a-world-war-ii-gi/.

CHAPTER 19

132 **the "high-tech," modern way to work out:** Bill Dobbins, *"High Tech" Training* (New York: Simon and Schuster, 1982), https://archive.org/details/hightechtraining00dobb.

133 **"NFR machines may be useful":** Yuri Verkhoshansky and Mel Siff, *Supertraining*, 6th ed. (Verkhoshansky.com, 2009), 238–9.

CHAPTER 20

137 **prevents them from just going and going and going forever:** Anson Rabinbach, *The Human Motor* (Berkeley: University of California Press, 1992), 35–36.

137 **whole institutions dedicated to measuring and understanding the contours and limits of human energy:** Anson Rabinbach, *The Human Motor* (Berkeley: University of California Press, 1992), 137.

138 **Reichardt had badly exaggerated the effects of his alleged vaccine:** Anson Rabinbach, *The Human Motor* (Berkeley: University of California Press, 1992), 143–4.

138 **but they only delayed an eventual even worse collapse:** Anson Rabinbach, *The Human Motor* (Berkeley: University of California Press, 1992), 144–5.

142 **between two people who are about the same size:** Nana Chung et al., "Non-exercise Activity Thermogenesis (NEAT): A Component of Total Daily Energy Expenditure," *Journal of Exercise Nutrition & Biochemistry* 22, no. 2 (2018): 23–30, https://doi.org/10.20463/jenb.2018.0013.

142 **is down to how much lean mass we have:** Chaitanya K. Gavini et al., "Leanness and Heightened Nonresting Energy Expenditure: Role of Skeletal Muscle Activity Thermogenesis," *American Journal of Physiology-Endocrinology and Metabolism* 306, no. 6 (2014): E635–47, https://doi.org/10.1152/ajpendo.00555.2013.

142 **a number of biological, genetic, and even environmental factors:** Nana Chung et al., "Non-exercise Activity Thermogenesis (NEAT): A Component of Total Daily Energy Expenditure," *Journal of Exercise Nutrition & Biochemistry* 22, no. 2 (2018): 23–30, https://doi.org/10.20463/jenb.2018.0013.

CHAPTER 21

147 **they can respond by disconnecting from their bodies in anticipation of getting hurt:** Judith Lewis Herman, *Trauma and Recovery: The Aftermath of Violence—From Domestic Abuse to Political Terror*, 4th ed. (New York: Basic Books, 2022), 54, Kindle.

148 **This field is called "interoception":** David Robson, "Interoception: The Hidden Sense That Shapes Wellbeing," *The Guardian*, August 15, 2021, https://www.theguardian

.com/science/2021/aug/15/the-hidden-sense-shaping-your-wellbeing-interoception.

149 **shares many symptoms with what is now known as dysautonomia:** M. J. Reichgott, "Clinical Evidence of Dysautonomia," chap. 76 in *Clinical Methods: The History, Physical, and Laboratory Examinations*, ed. H. K. Walker et al., 3rd ed. (Boston: Butterworths, 1990), https://www.ncbi.nlm.nih.gov/books/NBK400/.

149 **our ability to think clearly and make choices consistent with our values is related to our ability to attune and connect to our physical selves**: A.R. Damasio et al., "The Somatic Marker Hypothesis and the Possible Functions of the Prefrontal Cortex [and Discussion]," *Philosophical Transactions of the Royal Society B: Biological Sciences* 351, no. 1346 (1996): 1413–1420, https://doi.org/10.1098/rstb.1996.0125.

149 **People with anorexia, one study found, have particularly poor interoception:** Olga Pollatos et al., "Reduced Perception of Bodily Signals in Anorexia Nervosa," *Eating Behaviors* 9, no. 4 (2008): 381–88, https://doi.org/10.1016/j.eatbeh.2008.02.001.

150 **it also means we are unable to be truly present:** David Emerson and Elizabeth Hopper, *Overcoming Trauma Through Yoga* (Berkeley, CA: North Atlantic Books, 2011), 21–22, Kindle.

150 **"the avoidance or disregard of internal bodily experiences and the feeling of separateness from one's own body":** Marius Schmitz et al., "The Impact of Traumatic Childhood Experiences on Interoception: Disregarding One's Own Body," *Borderline Personality Disorder and Emotion Dysregulation* 10, no. 1 (2023): https://doi.org/10.1186/s40479-023-00212-5.

151 **increased brain-derived neurotrophic factor levels, and a few other processes:** Jill Kays et al., "The Dynamic Brain: Neuroplasticity and Mental Health," *Journal of Neuropsychiatry and Clinical Neurosciences* 24, no. 2 (2012): 118–24, https://doi.org/10.1176/appi.neuropsych.12050109.

151 **People with post-traumatic stress (particularly chronic stress):** Kim Eun Joo et al., "Stress Effects on the Hippocampus: A Critical Review," *Learning & Memory* 22, no. 9 (2015): 411–16, https://doi.org/10.1101/lm.037291.114.

151 **the authors specifically named malnutrition as a factor in lower hippocampal volume:** Enrico Collantoni et al., "Hippocampal Volumes in Anorexia Nervosa at Different Stages of the Disorder," *European Eating Disorders Review* 29, no. 1 (2020): 112–22, https://doi.org/10.1002/erv.2806.

151 **that was correlated with higher perceived stress:** Nathalie T. Burkert et al., "Structural Hippocampal Alterations, Perceived Stress, and Coping Deficiencies in Patients with Anorexia Nervosa," *International Journal of Eating Disorders* 48, no. 6 (2015): 670–76. https://doi.org/10.1002/eat.22397.

151 **when those anorexics recover, their hippocampal volume can recover:** Enrico Collantoni et al., "Hippocampal Volumes in Anorexia Nervosa at Different Stages of the Disorder," *European Eating Disorders Review* 29, no. 1 (2020): 112–22, https://doi.org/10.1002/erv.2806.

151 **food restriction can literally, biologically mess with the part of the brain:** Enrico

Collantoni et al., "The Hippocampus in Anorexia Nervosa," in *Eating Disorders*, ed. V. Patel and V. Preedy (Cham, Switzerland: Springer, 2023), 1–14, https://doi.org/10.1007/978-3-030-67929-3_30-1.

151 **strength training, in particular, is correlated with improved cognition:** R. C. Cassilhass et al., "Resistance Exercise Improves Hippocampus-Dependent Memory," *Brazilian Journal of Medical and Biological Research* 45, no. 12 (2012): 1215–20, https://doi.org/10.1590/s0100-879x2012007500138.

151 **it's also correlated with an increase in hippocampus volume:** Kim Yun Sik et al., "The Effects of Strength Exercise on Hippocampus Volume and Functional Fitness of Older Women," *Experimental Gerontology* 97 (October 2017): 22–28, https://doi.org/10.1016/j.exger.2017.07.007.

CHAPTER 22

157 **"feelings and sensations that arise from it as and when they do (not after or before)":** Laura Khoudari, *Lifting Heavy Things* (LifeTree Media, 2021), 13, Kindle.

158 **that the world around us is not real, or both:** "Depersonalization-Derealization Disorder," Mayo Clinic, May 16, 2017, https://www.mayoclinic.org/diseases-conditions/depersonalization-derealization-disorder/symptoms-causes/syc-20352911.

158 **"engaging more actively in the world":** Judith Lewis Herman, *Trauma and Recovery: The Aftermath of Violence—From Domestic Abuse to Political Terror*, 4th ed. (New York: Basic Books, 2022), 197, Kindle.

158 **"their traditional complicity in a hierarchy of dominance":** Judith Lewis Herman, *Trauma and Recovery: The Aftermath of Violence—From Domestic Abuse to Political Terror*, 4th ed. (New York: Basic Books, 2022), 197–9, Kindle.

160 **greater "self-esteem, risk detection, competence and a decrease in conflict sensitivity":** Margee Kerr and Linda Rodriguez, *Ouch! Why Pain Hurts, and Why It Doesn't Have To* (London: Bloomsbury Sigma, 2021), 148.

160 **it can lead to pain "catastrophizing":** Laura Petrini et al., "Understanding Pain Catastrophizing: Putting Pieces Together," *Frontiers in Psychology* 11, no. 1 (2020): https://doi.org/10.3389/fpsyg.2020.603420.

160 **based on how much pain they are experiencing:** Sarah Weiss et al., "On the Interaction of Self-Regulation, Interoception and Pain Perception," *Psychopathology* 47, no. 6 (2014): 377–82, https://doi.org/10.1159/000365107.

160 **"They've learned how to negotiate with pain…They take control":** Margee Kerr and Linda Rodriguez, *Ouch! Why Pain Hurts, and Why It Doesn't Have To* (London: Bloomsbury Sigma, 2021), 183.

161 **when people with arthritis received treatment for the "psychosocial" aspects, from experiencing anxiety and helplessness to maintaining leisure activities:** Catherine Backman, "Arthritis and Pain: Psychosocial Aspects in the Management of Arthritis Pain," *Arthritis Research and Therapy 8*, no. 221 (2006): https://doi.org/10.1186/ar2083.

CHAPTER 23

171 **"increasing cognitive abilities" by consuming antifungal dye meant for cleaning fish tanks:** Andrew Court, "Doctors Slam Influencers for Ingesting Fish Tank Cleaner to Fight Aging," *New York Post*, March 14, 2022, https://nypost.com/2022/03/14/doctors-slam-influencers-for-injecting-fish-tank-cleaner-to-fight-aging/.

171 **which she sold in 2021 for $400 million:** Andrew Michelson, "The World's Top Fitness Influencer Whose Instagram-Based 'Bikini Body Guide' Made Her a Millionaire Has Sold Her Empire for $400m," *Insider*, July 13, 2021, https://www.insider.com/worlds-top-fitness-influencer-kayla-itsines-sells-empire-sweat-400m-2021-7.

171 **her client testimonials on Instagram triggered, hastened, and worsened the onset of their eating disorders and body dysmorphia:** Giuseppe Tauriello, "Kayla Itsines, Tobi Pearce Join Forces to Take Back Ownership of Sweat," *The Advertiser*, November 21, 2023, https://www.adelaidenow.com.au/business/kayla-itsines-tobi-pearce-join-forces-to-take-back-ownership-of-sweat/news-story/769341f516cc0958c032e338d0e68b3e.

172 **damaging their physical and mental health and sending some of them to treatment:** Emily Olle, "Mother Says Daughter Developed Obsessive-Compulsive Disorder After Using Kayla Itsines' Bikini Body Guide," *The Advertiser*, May 9, 2022, https://www.adelaidenow.com.au/lifestyle/mother-says-daughter-developed-obsessivecompulsive-disorder-after-using-kayla-itsines-bikini-body-guide/news-story/7b9ef605da4cd01f3e73039231e0baea.

CHAPTER 24

176 **"powerlifters should train more like bodybuilders":** Greg Nuckols, "Powerlifters Should Train More like Bodybuilders," Stronger by Science, February 8, 2015, https://www.strongerbyscience.com/powerlifters-should-train-more-like-bodybuilders/.

179 **Mickey Rourke claimed to gain twenty-seven pounds of muscle in six months:** Michael Allen Smith, "How Mickey Rourke Gained 27 Pounds of Muscle for the Wrestler—Critical MAS," Critical MAS, January 7, 2009, https://criticalmas.org/2009/01/how-mickey-rourke-gained-27-pounds-of-muscle-for-the-wrestler/.

179 **Emma Stone's trainer claimed she gained 15 pounds of muscle in three months for *Battle of the Sexes*:** Carly Mallenbaum, "Here's How Emma Stone Gained 15 Pounds (of Muscle) for 'Battle of the Sexes,'" *USA TODAY*, September 25, 2017, https://www.usatoday.com/story/life/entertainthis/2017/09/24/heres-how-emma-stone-gained-15-pounds-of-muscle-battle-sexes/691127001/.

179 **Gal Gadot claimed to gain 17 pounds of muscle in nine months for *Batman v Superman: Dawn of Justice*:** Douglas Parkes, "Gal Gadot, Demi Moore and 3 Other Hollywood Actresses Who Got Ripped for Movie Roles," *South China Morning Post*, February 24, 2020, https://www.scmp.com/magazines/style/news-trends/article/3051816/gal-gadot-demi-moore-and-3-other-hollywood-actresses.

CHAPTER 25

184 **in an effort to protect them from further damage:** G. Greogry Haff and N. Travis Triplett, *Essential Principles of Strength Training*, 4th ed. (Champaign, IL: Human Kinetics, 2016), 94.

CHAPTER 28

203 **it's the fastest process for building muscle that exists:** Even though I used cutting and bulking, and cutting and bulking seems to work pretty well for most people, it's not the only way. Part of the reason cutting follows bulking, in theory, is that carrying extra body fat was thought to inhibit the muscle-gaining process. But there is some research that suggests body fat is not as interruptive to muscle building as the bro scientists previously thought. There is also the idea that muscle doesn't need to be built as efficiently as possible, unless you discover some kind of elite talent and are rushing your way to nationals, the Olympics, and sponsorships. Eric Trexler and Greg Nuckols, "Body-Fat and P-Ratios: A Rebuttal to the Rebuttal," Stronger by Science, March 2, 2021, https://www.strongerbyscience.com/p-ratios-rebuttal/.

204 **Body fat stores vitamins:** Rachel Crowley, "What Do Fats Do in the Body?," *Biomedical Beat Blog*, National Institute of General Medical Sciences, January 24, 2024, https://biobeat.nigms.nih.gov/2024/01/what-do-fats-do-in-the-body/.

204 **and regulates hormones, including estrogen, insulin, and cortisol:** "Body Fat," The Nutrition Source, Harvard T. H. Chan School of Public Health, August 2022, https://www.hsph.harvard.edu/nutritionsource/healthy-weight/measuring-fat/.

204 **Certain immune cells found in fat are even anti-inflammatory:** "Body Fat," The Nutrition Source, Harvard T. H. Chan School of Public Health, August 2022, https://www.hsph.harvard.edu/nutritionsource/healthy-weight/measuring-fat/.

205 **In one of her "peak week" videos:** Nikki Blackketter, "Peak Week | Grocery Haul & Scoping Out the Competition," YouTube, July 12, 2015, https://www.youtube.com/watch?v=hdIxRGgQqoY.

205 **In a video from the day before the competition:** Nikki Blackketter, "The Final Update | 1 Day Out," YouTube, July 21, 2015, https://www.youtube.com/watch?v=a79X1MAuu6M.

205 **"I don't think when you're that lean it's actually healthy for you":** Lisa Respers France, "Channing Tatum Deems Training for 'Magic Mike 3' as 'Unhealthy,'" CNN, February 22, 2022, https://www.cnn.com/2022/02/22/entertainment/channing-tatum-magic-mike-unhealthy/index.html.

206 **"they're either psychotic or unemployed, because it is a full time job":** Cori Ritchey, "Eric André Lost Nearly 40 Pounds to Disguise Himself. Here's How He Did It," *Men's Health*, June 2, 2023, https://www.menshealth.com/entertainment/a44077513/eric-andre-weight-loss/.

CHAPTER 29

210 **it was now written into my DNA:** David R. Jones et al., "Nucleus Type-Specific DNA Methylomics Reveals Epigenetic 'Memory' of Prior Adaptation in Skeletal Muscle," *Function* 2, no. 5 (2021): https://doi.org/10.1093/function/zqab038.

210 **"Why Women Can't Do Pull-Ups":** Tara Parker-Pope, "Why Women Can't Do Pull-Ups," *New York Times*, October 25, 2012, https://archive.nytimes.com/well.blogs.nytimes.com/2012/10/25/why-women-cant-do-pull-ups/.

210 **as if they were just smaller men with more biological complications, like menstruation:** G. Thomas et al., "Why Women Are Not Small Men: Sex-Related Differences in Perioperative Cardiopulmonary Exercise Testing," *Perioperative Medicine* 9, no. 1 (2020): https://doi.org/10.1186/s13741-020-00148-2.

211 **women tend to start losing muscle (as well as bone mass):** Kazuhiro Ikeda et al., "Functions of Estrogen and Estrogen Receptor Signaling on Skeletal Muscle," *Journal of Steroid Biochemistry and Molecular Biology* 191, July (2019): 105375, https://doi.org/10.1016/j.jsbmb.2019.105375.

211 **one of the best ways to augment a decline in estrogen in order to protect muscle was—you guessed it—exercise:** Andrea Pellegrino et al., "Mechanisms of Estrogen Influence on Skeletal Muscle: Mass, Regeneration, and Mitochondrial Function," *Sports Medicine* 52 (July 2022): https://doi.org/10.1007/s40279-022-01733-9.

211 **Women's strength and muscle size are often compared unfavorably to men's:** A. E. J. Miller et al., "Gender Differences in Strength and Muscle Fiber Characteristics," *European Journal of Applied Physiology and Occupational Physiology* 66, no. 3 (1993): 254–62, https://doi.org/10.1007/bf00235103.